Taking Care of
People with
DEMENTIA

An A-Z of practical help
and caregivers' stories

JE Hardacre. RMN. SRN.

CW00551898

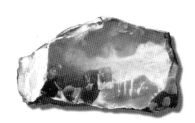

St Luke's Queen's Park Press

CREDITS

British Library Catalogue in Publication Data
A catalogue record for this book is available from the British Library
ISBN 978-0-9934041-2-2

First published in Great Britain in 2017 by St Luke's Queen's Park Press, Brighton, Great Britain

TYPESET	Woking Print & Publicity
DESIGNER	Richard Woods
MANAGING EDITOR	Julie Newson
EDITOR	Evlynn Sharp
PHOTOGRAPHER	Evlynn Sharp, Images © 2017
PRINTED AND BOUND	Woking Print & Publicity, The Print Works, St John's Lye, Woking, Surrey GU21 1RS Tel: 01483 884884

DEDICATION

For carers and people with dementia everywhere, for my beloved son, and my dear mum.

" *In the midst of any situation, the qualities of sincerity, kindness and empathy are the precious resource we share as human beings – speaking from the heart of our lives, listening to each other's way of survival, sharing our experiences, our personal hardships and our hopes.* "

– JE Hardacre

ACKNOWLEDGEMENTS

I offer my deepest thanks to everyone who has contributed towards this book in so many kind ways. To carers at home and people with dementia, carers who work in care homes, doctors and nurses in hospitals and other specialist staff in the medical profession, in charities, institutions, establishments.

My heart-felt gratitude especially to the Reverend Julie Newson for her support in the development of this book, and to the congregation of St Luke's Church, Queen's Park, Brighton, for their encouragement.

I am especially grateful to Ans Epskamp, Howard Rush, Joe Hughes, Stephanie Smith, Asha Small, Susannah Donovan, Rachel Dias who read through drafts of this book giving very supportive feedback.

My thanks for feedback on the book to all the other people and charities that prefer not to be named. Also, with grateful thanks to Evlynn Sharp for her wealth of knowledge, her editing, her patience and faith in me.

My great gratitude goes to my family and friends who have supported me throughout the writing of this book and encouraged me to keep going during times I felt like giving up.

I wish to thank Care for the Carers, the Carers Centre for East Sussex, a tremendous charity whose staff, values and work are inspirational. I particularly thank Teresa Flower, Strategic Partnerships Manager, and Grace Scrimgeour who set up a book club event where my book could be discussed. For information, please see: *www.cftc.org.uk*

Among others who attended the book club event, I would like to thank James Patmore for his sensitive comments and reflections, and Stephen Pett, Client Services Director, The Probate Department Ltd., Solicitors, also known as Eastbourne Law, for his valuable contribution.

– JE Hardacre

CONTENTS

INTRODUCTION

Taking Care of People with Dementia: an A-Z of practical help and caregivers' stories is about the realities of caring for individuals with dementia in its many forms.

The book presents practical hints, tips, advice and information for carers, for those who may become caregivers, and for all who would welcome insight into caring for those with dementia. It features personal reflections by carers on their feelings and experiences, which they hope create understanding and reveal what to expect in caregiving.

Dementia has become an umbrella term for different diseases and disorders that cause the condition. When dementia is mentioned, some might think about it as memory loss, the deterioration of a person's mental and physical condition, mainly in regard to elderly people.

But dementia occurs in individuals of all ages – and can go undiagnosed in younger people or those who may have a disability. Without testing, it will be unknown what type of dementia a person has and how this presents.

Types of dementia include Alzheimer's disease, which usually starts by affecting people's short-term memory. Another type can be caused when a major stroke or strokes have occurred – although not all lead to dementia as it depends on the location and severity of the stroke.

A carer whose wife's diagnosis is dementia with Lewy bodies (DLB) describes her as having memory loss and Parkinson's-like symptoms such as slow rigid movements, periods of alertness, restlessness and sleep disturbances.

Carers observe in Frontotemporal dementia – also called Pick's disease – how an individual's personality changes before any memory loss. Some people notice the risk of getting dementia seems to increase by excessive and continuous alcohol consumption.

Knowing the type of dementia will determine the form of treatment and support that is necessary. The progress from diagnosis to the time when a person is no longer able to self-care can take several years.

In the early stages of the illness, people may live well and independently in society. Businesses and banks may employ specialists to assist individuals with the condition whilst they are still fairly independent.

The nature of the disease brings about change, and *Taking Care of People with Dementia* addresses the emotional and practical needs of those who are passing the stage of living well with the disease into a state of high dependence – whose care needs may reach the point where caregivers can struggle to cope or to know about the complexity of providing care.

There is a growing cultural awareness of dementia through research and education. For people with dementia and for carers, there are excellent associations, organisations, societies, groups, initiatives and charities offering guidance, understanding, networking and help such as Care for the Carers in East Sussex and the Alzheimer's Society's Dementia Friends programme.

Carers deserve to be acknowledged in their caring roles – the work they do can be emotionally and physically demanding. Some carers reflect they feel uninformed, frustrated, taken for granted or used as cheap labour.

While improvements in support of people with dementia and carers have been made over time, among issues that remain the same include the fact that carers provide essential care. The number of people diagnosed with dementia is apparently on the increase, which implies more carers will be vital.

Through speaking like it is, *Taking Care of People with Dementia* represents the everyday challenges of caregiving and hopefully empowers people through wider knowledge.

This book is dedicated to all people with dementia – and to the incredible, courageous, loving and compassionate people who are their carers.

JE Hardacre, RMN, SRN, CPN
August 2017

FOREWORD

> "This is a book which is written for a lay person although many professionals would profit from being aware of its content and purpose. When my wife was initially diagnosed with dementia with Lewy bodies I needed to know exactly what was involved. It is a life-changing event for both the patient but more importantly the significant loved one, be they partner, relative or friend. Contact with the consultant or other knowledgeable health professional is limited in terms of time and availability... those individuals will be speaking in a highly technical language, which may, or may not, be fully understood by the recipient."

— James P, Carer

CHAPTER 1 — INDIVIDUALS

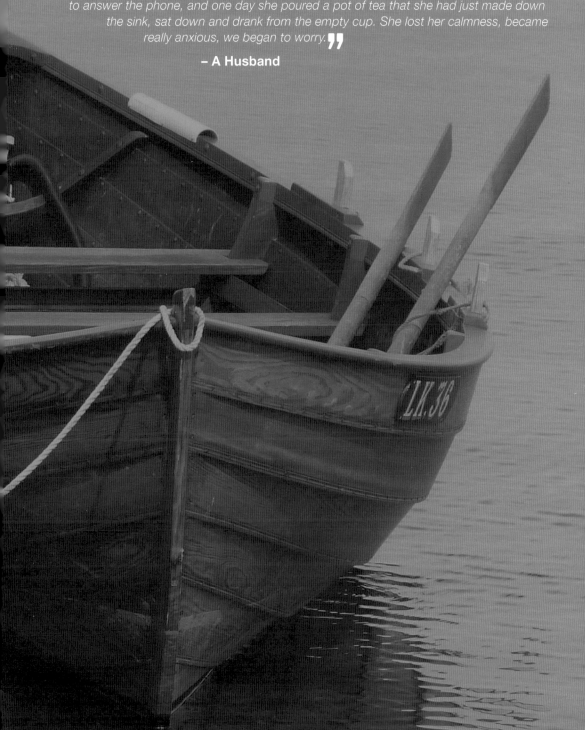

"My wife started forgetting things, everyday routines, names. We put it down to old age and laughed it off. Little by little other oddities were creeping in, like she would pick up the notepad to answer the phone, and one day she poured a pot of tea that she had just made down the sink, sat down and drank from the empty cup. She lost her calmness, became really anxious, we began to worry."

– A Husband

Every person with dementia was free of this condition once. No matter what the circumstances, dementia can take away from the peace and freedom in people's lives. The effects of this condition impact differently on the person with dementia and on the carer.

The emotional pain felt by individuals with dementia and carers may at times seem unbearable. People might not understand the how and why of dementia.

The background of those who exhibit the characteristics of dementia goes across age, race, class, gender. Some people may have occupied professional positions at work. Others may have spent their lives working in the home.

People with dementia may live with relatives. Some live alone. Some live with a partner. Some may still be actively working and enduring the stress and strain of trying to maintain a lifestyle which is slipping away. Some have their own family with children who may be quite young.

Carers whose husbands or wives are no longer functioning at their best might find the condition hard to take. Other carers may say a partner is no longer the person they knew, and that causes great sadness in them.

Sons and daughters of people living with dementia might no longer recognise the new personality of the parent as the dementia takes over. As people change, and independence and abilities are lost, then a son or daughter may find the role of carer hard to accept.

Carers – unpaid and paid – do their best to look after people with dementia who choose to remain in their own homes in an attempt to retain their independence and individuality.

Care homes and hospitals endeavour to treat the person with dementia with dignity and respect no matter how many other patients are showing similar signs, symptoms and behaviours.

Individuals deserve care, appreciation, respect, compassion, empathy and support to get through the reality of either living with dementia or caring for others with the condition.

> **"***Tho' much is taken, much abides; and tho'***
> ***We are not now that strength which in old days***
> ***Moved earth and heaven, that which we are, we are...***"**
>
> – **Extract from *Ulysses* by Alfred, Lord Tennyson**

CHAPTER 2 — ONSET

"I fell out with my mum first and then my sister. I used to go round to my mum's in the early stages before she got put into a home. She started to accuse me of taking her purse. We'd look for it together; when we found it she would go through it as if she expected to find money missing. Reasoning never worked. My mum told my sister someone was taking money from her purse; as no one else but me visited, my sister decided to believe her. The fact that money was found stowed away in various places all over the house when she left, did nothing to reconcile our relationship."

– A Daughter

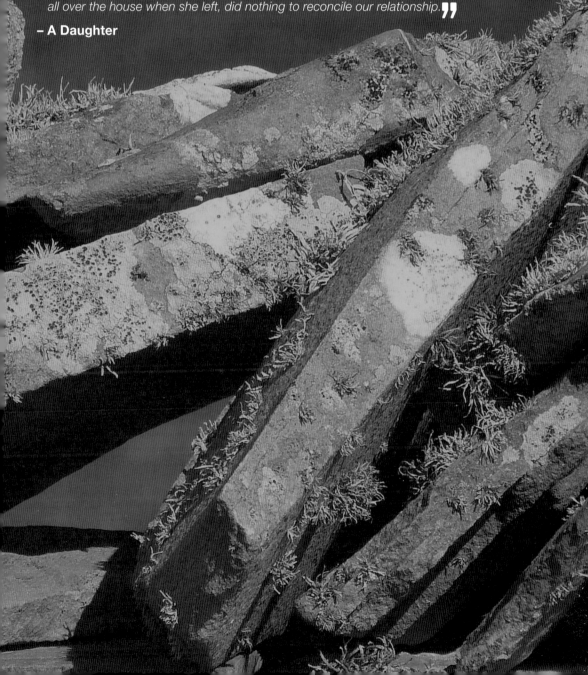

> ❝I couldn't believe it when my nan told me she'd made friends with a lovely young couple who do all kinds of things for her. My nan is a very friendly old lady who doesn't believe she's 77. She still thinks that she's back in the days of her youth. She told me they got her shopping for her, they put it away, did cleaning for her, made sure she ate her meals and everything. She wasn't lonely because they came round every evening to watch telly with her and enjoyed the take-away meals. When I asked her who paid for the shopping and meals she said they did because they had her pension book which they cashed every week for her, and it was only fair as they did so much for her. She'd no idea where her pension book was and how much money she had in her account.❞
>
> – **A Granddaughter**

The beginning of the journey into dementia can take between two and five years before anyone realises what is happening. Some types of dementia are difficult to differentiate – one can present like another, and if the person has suffered a stroke or a series of little strokes, there may be periods of improvement and people can think everything is going to be alright.

The signs will be there, though. At first forgetfulness may be passed off as old age, and becomes a family joke, but the person's memory does not come back. And as it progresses the person facing the onset of dementia has to keep being reminded of familiar faces, places and events.

This loss of memory may lead to depression as the person can be aware of what is happening as well as being prone to paranoia, suspicion and accusations.

Individuals with the early onset of dementia can become increasingly upset and fearful and people begin to be careful of what is said around them for fear of making them worse.

One type of dementia results in the person forgetting a word or making up words when the correct word is forgotten. This practice can cause humour in those around and be seen as a quirky thing that happens – but as it continues, it stops being funny. After a while, the speaking stops.

Lack of inhibition in someone who is shy or formal begins to take hold. A person with the onset of dementia can become flirty, expose themselves, use swear words or expressions of a lewd nature they would never have uttered before. People can become argumentative and may refuse to admit there is something amiss.

Other signs that reveal the onset of dementia include the failure to complete basic tasks around the home – even simple tasks become a challenge. Household gadgets are mistaken for other objects and people can forget how to use them.

> ❝I once worked with a woman who was diagnosed with young onset dementia. She was fifty-five. She presented with memory impairment, and an inability to maintain and carry out her activities of daily living in varying degrees. It was difficult for her family to recognise she was on the way to dementia so advice was sought late. As far as they were concerned she was young, seemed fit, and she was continuing with her working life to some extent.❞
>
> – **Staff Nurse in an Assessment Unit**

Leaving home very late at night or going to attend an activity that took place years ago are common signs of dementia. Mobility starts to be affected, and as carers become fearful about people's safety they worry about leaving them on their own.

People who have been meticulous about their clothing and looks can experience loss of interest in personal appearance or hygiene. Also, people may speak about someone who passed away as if the person is still alive. Or they might ask the same question repeatedly as if not satisfied with the answer and are forgetful they asked the question.

The onset of dementia in people can change the behaviour of those around them. Relatives, parents, friends, or other carers might find neither strength nor patience to cope. Sadness, feelings of hopelessness, exasperation and hostility can begin to take hold in carers as well as feelings of being put upon.

A-Z and reflections for carers

Advice at the start – needs to be sought early as soon as signs of behaviour appear that is out of character and cause concern so that infections, constipation, drug reactions, depression, a brain tumour, and other reasons for the confused and distressing behaviour can be ruled out. Not all confusion means the onset of dementia, and it is wise to seek an early opinion. Not all memory loss is due to dementia, and with regular testing of memory and verbal ability, it could be easier for a doctor to spot decline or changes and rule out other diseases or causes that may be treatable.

"*My dad went downhill after our mum died. At first we thought it was just grief, which was understandable as they'd been married for over 50 years. But he rallied and each of us took it in turn to make sure he had Sunday lunch with one of us and we invited him to all family events and birthday parties. He continued to play golf, he was a keen cricketer, even going to away matches for weekends with the team. That was alright for the first five years after mum died but about two years on…he'd forget some words and make up others to take their place and laugh about it, he'd say, 'You know what I mean.' He would start the journey to our house but would end up in the supermarket and when asked why he did that he'd make an excuse and say as far as he was concerned nothing had been really planned, he felt he could do as he pleased. He never became stroppy but we knew when to leave a subject alone. That period of forgetfulness went on for quite a while with no other alarm bells ringing for us; he continued to live on his own with a neighbour popping in and everyone made allowances for him. Matters got worse in terms of him being safe; we'd notice when we went round the pans were burnt, kitchen towels were scorched, his accumulation of papers and stuff was making it a hazard he could trip over or a fire risk. He was still driving and we asked the GP about it; but because he'd not had an accident and kept to the same routes the doctor said to let him continue for a bit longer. It came to a head when a member of his club asked us about a female companion with whom dad had been regularly seen. He said she was a friend who was down on her luck, recently in the area, he was befriending her. Very soon after when I went round to see him, she was in the house and claimed she was living there. My sisters had never seen her on their visits, leading us to suspect she had been hiding or they had missed her when she visited. Despite all of us reasoning with dad and suggesting the woman was not all she claimed to be, he allowed her to stay with him. Worst of all she slept in his bed while he slept on the settee; he waited on her hand and foot and spent a lot of money on her.*

He spent no money on himself and instead of being the dapper man we knew, he became less clean and less bothered about himself. He accused us of being worried about his Will and not his welfare. He refused to see the GP again because the woman told him he didn't need to; he's stopped coming round to us. We only see him now when we go round. He was enjoying this new experience and refused to be turned away from it. Because he won't see the doctor or any professional, we are unsure as to the state of his mind…is that the start of things? **"**

– A Daughter

Denial – can be one of the factors why the onset of dementia is not recognised and treated. If an attitude or behaviour begins to cause concern, then action should be taken to ascertain the cause. It is crucial to be vigilant and look for early signs of the onset. Denial can prevent proper early diagnosis and care.

"*It was embarrassing. The police came to the door to return our dad. We thought he was asleep upstairs and to tell you the truth we were relieved he had settled down as he had been fidgeting all day, moving and tidying everything. They'd found him wandering the streets nearby and had no idea who he was or where he lived, and he only avoided spending the night in hospital because a neighbour recognised him. My dad was in his pyjamas and would've been mortified if he was aware of what was going on. We were trying to keep his decreasing mental health a secret from our neighbours but now we could do that no longer; it was a wake-up call for us.* **"**

– A Daughter

People sometimes fob off behaviour with unhelpful statements that suggest the person with dementia was always a bit 'loopy' or never remembered the grandchildren's names anyway. Or a person may have been labelled a picky eater. Yet within eighteen months to two years from the onset of dementia people can start to look skeletal, and weight loss is apparent – although they claim to be eating.

Also, people with dementia can spend their money on useless gadets they have seen in newspapers, magazines or elsewhere. Money is given away to all and sundry including as a result of scam calls and letters. Medication prescribed may not be taken even although a person swears compliance.

Depression – often thought of as being part of ageing and dementia and is therefore not considered in its own right. There may be a good reason for depression and proper treatment is able to restore health. It is worth pushing for treatment for possible depression rather than accepting judgements that some old people behave a certain way and are apathetic, weepy.

Some illnesses may look like dementia and can be cleared up with antibiotics, anti-depressants, high doses of vitamins, or even an anti-thyroid treatment. But it will be clear that something more is amiss when the person shows obvious signs of impending dementia.

Depression in people of a young age coupled with behavioural changes should be looked at closely.

Early detection and some treatments can slow down the process for a few years or months.

Ignorance – of dementia and how to cope can lead to abuse and injury of a carer and of the one being cared for. It is better to be in the know.

There are numerous support networks and organisations that can provide essential information to address particular needs such as the Alzheimer's Society, Carers UK, Age UK, Care for the Carers, and Dementia UK.

These organisations have significant experience, tactics of care and substantial knowledge of caring for people with dementia. Carers can have discussions with staff there and others such as care home employees and pass on information to each other, ideas about what works for them, and to let each other know how it feels to be listened to, and how to cope. For example, carers might find it difficult to look after people with dementia especially in the area of private intimate care. So it can be a relief to talk to professional staff and other carers about such problems.

Carers may use on-line networks to share and lighten their load, their anxieties, their fears, to share their guilt and mistakes, to make jokes that can help ease worries, and to share resources such as information.

Intelligence – do not assume people with the onset of dementia are also stupid. During occasions such as family gatherings, people with dementia may be resting yet listening. They may want to be more involved and included in discussions – or not. Or they may speak out unexpected statements or questions in the course of a family discussion, which would need a sensitive response.

> ❝*Mother asked a question! 'Is your sister still married to that b******?' She'd been sitting there quietly, almost forgotten during the family get-together at a relative's house. It was assumed she and a cousin were propping each other up and competing for sleep space on the settee, so the conversation about who is who, who is where, and who was doing what with whom was not whispered as there seemed to be no need. She made that statement or rather asked that question and was welcomed back into the conversation but then we lost her a little later when she retreated into her comfortable world of less exhausting attention.*❞

– A Daughter

Memory – starts to go about recent events and about what to do with items that have lost their familiarity. Life around begins to become unsafe. Past events may be discussed with some detail, but even then people experiencing the onset of dementia can be unaware they are speaking to a family member such as their son or daughter.

Speak out – carers may need determination to get health professionals to listen to, and take seriously, their concerns regarding the onset of dementia in a loved one. What helps is to put things down on paper, to reflect on what the person says or does or has stopped doing that is causing concern, especially if behavioural problems worsen.

Carers can record these issues for their GP and report side effects of any medications or treatments prescribed. Carers may need to be outspoken regarding the outcome of assessments and dates of reviews. If support is needed when speaking out and if face-to-face meetings are awkward, carers can nominate someone else to confront situations on their behalf.

People with dementia can be asked to attend a meeting of carers and others when decisions about their care are raised. They can be aware of what is being said around them but may be unable to verbally contribute.

Some people with dementia have no one to speak up for them. An Independent Mental Capacity Advocate (IMCA) can be appointed to act in the best interest of a person who is deemed not to have capacity.

Paranoia – people with dementia may feel everyone is plotting against them to do them harm. It is generally an unfounded fear but can be quite a dangerous condition.

By the time my father had worn my mother down with accusations and followed them up with physical assaults, his fears that he may be harmed by her had an element of truth. It had all been explained earlier to them that paranoia was a feature of dementia especially at the onset, and ran alongside the confusion and forgetfulness. Father repeatedly accused mother of hiding his wallet, his books, and his personal possessions and badgered her into owning up. Mother used to help look for the items but then she ran the risk of being hit when she did find them because it proved to him she had them all along! If she did not look for it, the day or part of the day was spent fending off answers to the constant questioning about the missing articles, with the house being turned upside down during the hunt. The search did not always take place during the day because some nights when he should have been sleeping he could be found rummaging through drawers looking for God knows what because he would not answer when she asked him. He accused her of being a thief and a liar and said she couldn't be trusted. Several cups of tea and soothing words later he may be led back to bed and the whole incident would be forgotten by the morning. This was repeated at other times and occasionally with worse effects. Mother was pushed down the stairs by father in one of these paranoid rages and it was then that the family decided she could no longer look after him without threat of injury to herself, so sadly a home had to be found for him.

– A Daughter

Question – if hospital admission is required by people with dementia for any reason, carers need to question why certain treatments are offered or drugs are prescribed. Also, carers must question if treatments are not being followed up or why results of scans are taking a long time to come through.

Question if hospital staff are thinking of a discharge home and yet the individual does not seem ready, or the house is not prepared. In a care home, question apparent shortcomings in people's care.

Valuing and despairing – as dementia progresses, the more heartbreaking it can be for family carers and others to witness. Sometimes carers may feel so despairing they foster suicidal thoughts. In this instance, carers must seek professional help urgently.

Carers value people for whom they are providing care but may be struggling to cope. So there may be an underlying feeling to let people die with dignity before the illness totally takes over. Carers should always seek professional support to discuss such feelings and put adequate care in place for people with dementia.

Wisdom – it may be a good idea to have conversations about care and death whilst people are in good mental health and the threat of a debilitating illness or a progressive one such as dementia seems remote. People might say they do not want to end up like their mother or father or aunt in a care home. Whilst care homes have improved, old attitudes towards them may remain, and even some fear. Gain wisdom around choices about care that may need to be made.

Golden Rules

DO NOT hide people's behaviour from others in the family. There is no shame in having a loved one with dementia. People with dementia can wander off, start taking off their clothes in inappropriate places, start making up words in the middle of an ordinary conversation – so others will be aware of their condition anyway.

DO NOT cut off from people with dementia if they swear, or smell, or tell anyone who listens that their carer has stolen from them.

DO NOT go it alone. Try not to let your energy be sapped as this can put at risk personal well-being, vitality, and drain hope. When an emotional and behavioural change is apparent in a loved one, and action has been taken, then others involved may want to know what is happening.

DO NOT self-blame. Nothing will change the situation of dementia onset. People must not blame themselves by thinking they should have seen the dementia coming or acted sooner.

DO NOT forget to inform the Driver and Vehicle Licensing Agency (DVLA) if a person has been diagnosed with dementia.

DO NOT be afraid to find out about dementia. Carers doing research on all types of dementia have been helped to understand what people go through. This inquiry is important in relation to young people as they may present differently from older people. Fears and curiosity are well-founded, and seeking out information by becoming involved in the assessment of a loved one's mental state can help to alleviate anxieties.

DO NOT be afraid of dementia. Although it seems daunting, carers' knowledge, attitude to and relationship with the individual are in their control.

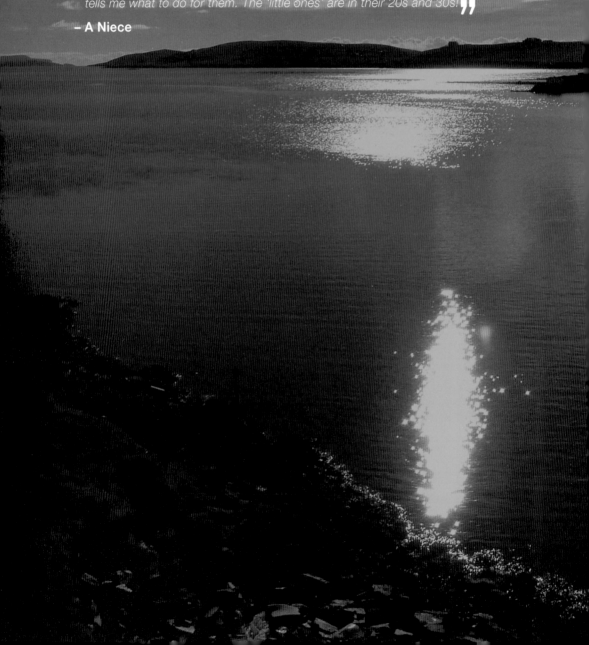

CHAPTER 3 — EARLY STAGES: SPECIALIST PEOPLE TO CONTACT

"They say if you don't use it you will lose it. That's not true. My aunt was a nanny and she travelled all over Europe, she can speak about six languages and was fluent in four of them. She has early stage dementia; still tries to converse when we speak to her in French or Italian but not as good as she was. She can just about manage English sensibly. She still thinks she's looking after the little ones, corrects their manners and tells me what to do for them. The 'little ones' are in their 20s and 30s!"

– A Niece

Carers can research and discover the process involved in determining a person's dementia. Symptoms present early and are among the key factors in suspecting and diagnosing early onset of the condition. The memory loss in dementia interferes with everyday activities resulting in confusion and forgetfulness.

Assessment

GPs take a personal history of the patient examining lifestyle factors such as smoking, excessive alcohol consumption, also strokes, heart disease, and other clues that may determine the type of dementia that is likely to be present. Also, GPs may take a history of family to establish if there is someone or has been someone in the family with dementia. In looking to identify dementia, a GP may suggest blood tests to exclude vitamin deficiency, glandular disorders, diabetes, hypertension or an infection.

In one type of assessment, the examination is based on a series of tests known as the Mini Mental State Examination (MMSE). The GP – or the assessor – will ask basic questions, ask the patient to recite a sequence of numbers, or, among other tasks, to repeat a statement made, or to copy a drawing. The MMSE has a score attached so the GP, or assessor, will determine where along the scale the patient has scored. This score can give an indication of the brain's impairment. Memory clinics also perform similar tests that may lead to a diagnosis.

Assessment by MMSE is a demanding procedure and can reveal in people a lack of comprehension when an explanation has been given on a particular topic; the inability to keep track of what is being told; the inability to use an object for its purpose; vagueness in a familiar place; lack of recognition of familiar objects and pictures.

As dementia progresses, and this testing is repeated, a drop in the scoring will occur that denotes deterioration in the mental – cognitive – functioning, and impaired physical ability.

If people forget how to undertake a particular task or do not recognise an object they will not know what to do. So there is a decreasing ability of self-care such as basic tasks of hygiene.

Another type of examination requires information from relatives or carers about a person's sleeping or wakefulness habits, or incidences of hallucinations, particularly visual ones, and mood variations. This information can determine what type of dementia the person may be experiencing.

A-Z and reflections for carers

Once the presence of dementia is suspected and recognised, there can be many qualified people involved in care.

Care home manager – who may visit the person with dementia in hospital or at home. Care home managers can use this opportunity to meet people who may be admitted to their facility and will make a decision as to whether or not individuals will be best placed there.

Community psychiatric nurse (CPN) – who will mostly make home visits to ensure carers have not been abused by a person with dementia or vice versa, and that carers and individuals are coping as well as can be expected.

The CPN will be helpful to carers and those with dementia in assessing the effects of mental deterioration and offering support.

The CPN is also the person who can request an urgent placement either in a care home or hospital as someone's mental health deteriorates or if the carer is feeling overwhelmed, or is being threatened, or has an illness, or needs admission to hospital.

If people with dementia are living on their own, the CPN will ensure there is compliance if medication has been prescribed, and report back to the GP on people's mental and physical states.

Doctor – GPs can put carers in touch with a range of services such as care that is available in the community and with people including occupational therapists, social workers, and community psychiatric nurses. GPs will alert others to the needs of carers such as the necessity of home visits, delivery of prescriptions, or synchronicity of appointments.

Occupational therapist (OT) – visits people in their homes to assess the need for physical aids and practical improvements. OTs can also advise on the suitability of the home accommodation. They are able to take a long-term view of care requirements.

Social worker – carries out community care assessments in hospital or people's homes. Social workers along with others in the multi-disciplinary team have access to information about care establishments. Carers can be given a list of places that may be suitable or asked to check out places via the internet.

Golden Rules

MAKE DECISIONS early. If a carer wants to look after a person with dementia at home then the caregiver must become aware of resources available to support that decision and make choices about care provision.

FIND OUT through GPs how to contact health professionals who can offer help.

MAKE FRIENDS with local pharmacists as they have a wealth of knowledge. Pharmacies will deliver medication to people's homes. As long as prescriptions are kept updated as prescribed this service will help carers especially if circumstances such as weather or personal health make it difficult to go out.

ASSESS FINANCES to check if changes and adaptations to the home are required and funds can be put in place.

CHAPTER 4 — THE CARE PACKAGE

> " I used to take my wife two days a week for respite to a day centre, part of an assessment unit in the hospital. I felt very smug, she could travel with me and not have to be brought in by the minibus. I thought she was not like the others, she would never get like them. Together, we made sure she was smartly dressed, clean, well-fed. I didn't need help; my sons had their jobs and their families and didn't want to have to look after mum – that was what I was there for. This arrangement lasted almost two years; during that time she became dependent on me, and whereas before I could leave her in the house and pop down to the shops, it was becoming apparent I could no longer do that. She became quiet and weepy, sad and fearful, but wouldn't say why. After a while, I had to take her everywhere I went. She had stopped helping me to get herself dressed, she just sat there waiting for me to do it, even to put on her makeup. It came to a head one day when I left her strapped in the car while I unloaded the shopping and took it to our kitchen door. After the second trip I looked in the car and she was gone. When I looked down the road she was legging it and had almost reached the corner. The incident made me depressed – I thought I had it all under control. I frightened myself into thinking, what if she had crossed the road and got run over? I had to admit the respite care would have to turn into long-term care when I could no longer keep her safe. "

– A Husband

Carers will need to explore in their local area what is on offer for people with dementia and for themselves; the authorities may recommend people remain in their own home for as long as possible. In this way, people with dementia will be in an environment they recognise, be among relatives, friends and neighbours, and their own possessions, and feel involved in their regular social scene. But care needs differ. Also, what is available to caregivers and individuals with dementia can depend on where people live – such as the funding and accessibility of social care and other services, the variety of services and workforce.

> **"**A husband was admitted to hospital on account of what was thought of his onset of Alzheimer's causing emotional and physical harm to his wife. Whilst he was being assessed in the hospital, his wife suffered a stroke, brought on, apparently, by the stress of the whole thing. She was admitted to hospital. The plan was he'd be discharged with medication under the care of the GP and a community psychiatric nurse. When his wife was discharged via a rehab unit, she'd have a discharge plan in place that meant she'd receive the attention of a separate, appropriate care team at home. After a frank discussion, it was realised the situation couldn't work. The wife couldn't look after the husband as before and, taking into consideration his abusive behaviour, she was now more vulnerable; his dementia would only get worse. It was a very difficult decision for the family and the care team to make but the husband was placed in a care home, and live-in care staff was paid for his wife until such time as she was more able to take care of herself.**"**
>
> – **A Caregiver**

A-Z and reflections for carers

Care package – an arrangement between carers and the support team that aims to provide initial and follow-up care such as after an individual's discharge from hospital.

The care package can become complicated depending on the needs of individuals, for example, a couple became ill at the same time and required care at home following different discharge dates from the hospital.

Holiday – carers need to take a holiday as often as practicable.

A physical and emotional break is essential. Respite can be arranged with professional carers. Any anxieties and worry may be eased once carers know the person with dementia will be well looked after in their absence. Family members may be able to help out, even if only for a short time.

Personal assistant (PA)/community support worker (CSW) – provides care and support for people with dementia in their own home. Carers can advertise for PAs or CSWs or ask agencies.

All non-family support comes at a price. People need paying for their services – through direct payment from the carer who becomes their employer, or through an employment agency or health authority. Support workers must come with professional references and police checks through the Disclosure and Barring Service (DBS).

Respite care – a service provided by some care homes that will take in people with dementia over an agreed period, which allows the carer at home to have time off. It is possible to arrange with a home this kind of care with a view to people moving in permanently when they deteriorate. In this way, the care home and its staff will already be familiar with people's needs.

Golden Rules

TAKE UP OFFERS OF RESPITE as caregivers will not be letting themselves or others down if they admit to needing a break every now and then.

CHECK on the fee for the respite break offered by a care home, or by any other place. Carers may be able to receive financial assistance for their own break from the local council, depending on assessments.

SHOP AROUND for other carers or friends who can assist the primary carer in the day-to-day running of the household and in providing effective care for the person with dementia.

CHECK the credibility of any person such as social worker, personal assistant, community support worker and others allowed into the home. Check the DBS is current. If carers feel unable to do so, then ask someone else such as a family member to confirm the police check – DBS – is current.

DECISIONS TO CARE for a person with dementia at home is a kind gesture but may not have been made easy especially if others oppose this course. People with dementia may have been assessed as being able to live by themselves for a while, with family or others popping in regularly. However the decision comes about, care at home demands patience and understanding.

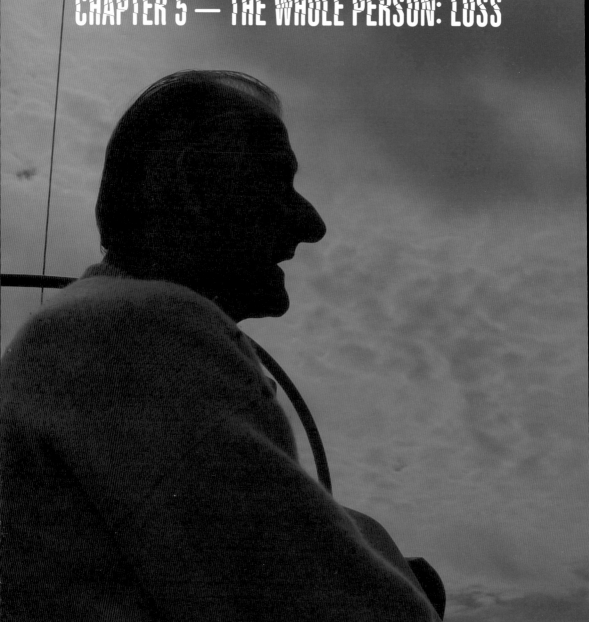

CHAPTER 5 — THE WHOLE PERSON: LOSS

Carers have to do for people with dementia what the brain has stopped doing, and think about what is necessary for those who depend on them. The scale of deterioration dementia brings about reflects that people have lost the part of their brain which enabled them to function all their lives.

A-Z and reflections for carers

"When you talk about the whole person, you should get a mental picture in your head of the person's body, working from their head to their toes."

– A Tutor

Loss of control of bodily functions – people with dementia may not be able to let people know when they want to use the toilet, or to know they need to use the toilet, or may not recognise they have done the toilet in their underwear.

Carers should try to establish a toilet routine for the person that prevents and pre-empts accidents. This practice means caregivers must closely observe people's body language, or listen out for noises, and in a care home must read about people's toileting routine and ensure it is carried out. It is not a nice feeling to a person or good for the skin to be sitting in urine or faecal matter for any length of time.

"If my resident with dementia isn't able to assist with the cleaning up process, I may need an extra pair of hands and a manual handling aid. If it's been decided that they'd be more protected by wearing a pad or incontinence pants of some sort, that's still no excuse to leave people in them for any length of time. I'll still need to promptly check to see if a person's pad or pants needs changing."

– Care Home Worker

Loss of hearing – this condition may be the deafness that can come with ageing or a slower response to what is heard. Carers will have to be people's ears and also act as a go-between to let others know if individuals have not heard or may not have understood.

Carers can take time to approach a person with dementia face-to-face to tell them what they are going to do or what someone else wants them to do. Shouting or speaking loudly does not help. Coming up on people suddenly can cause them to be frightened.

"It's important to let everyone involved in care know if my residents have a hearing problem. Otherwise someone might give a command to them, and then walk off expecting them to have heard, or to know what has been said and to obey it."

– Care Home Worker

Loss of memory – carers have to be the memory of a person with dementia. Play games that may remind people of themselves as a younger person, and remind them of the jobs they did. Play songs that reflect the age and era during which people lived. Show them personal pictures such as of a wife, a husband, or of a sister, a brother, or of their children and grandchildren. Make conversations that talk about people's younger days. Some days they will not know those close to them and will not remember a thing. Caregivers must be careful using these approaches to connect with the person just in case the activity sparks excessive weepiness.

Loss of reasoning – in care homes, carers may not be able to reason with someone who has dementia about why they cannot walk about naked, or to leave the premises. Also, carers may have to get permission to restrict people's freedom if the risk of someone's potential for self-harm is extreme. Carers may have to tell a person with dementia every day why they cannot do certain things.

Loss of sight – this condition is not always blindness in people with dementia, but loss of recognition of familiar objects, people and places, even of themselves. Carers may have to be like the eyes of a person with dementia. Carers may need to plan a colour scheme that helps the person to see the difference between objects.

Loss of speech – it is not known why some individuals with dementia stop speaking. In the early days carers may find people forgetting words, or making up words, or they themselves become embarrassed by the slowness of their response especially if they have had a stroke. Later, the effort of communication may result in a person not speaking at all.

Carers will have to be the voice of the person with dementia. If carers are based in a care home, they can read the admission notes and find out people's likes and dislikes, and about their background. This information is important in the caring of someone with dementia as the carer has to champion and communicate on another's behalf.

Also, carers will have to read people's eyes, face, and body language as this may be their only way of communicating what they would like.

If people with dementia can speak and mention pain, or their body language alerts to a problem, then it is a carer's responsibility to find relief for them.

> **"**I may get a nod of acknowledgement from my dementia resident, or a smile to let me know that the message has been received and understood, or I'll get a blank look staring at me. Either way, I always speak to her as if she will respond.**"**
>
> **– Care Home Worker**

Loss of swallowing reflex – some foods may be difficult to chew, or people might take a long time chewing. Carers must ensure people with dementia receive foods appropriate to their dental state, and are given time to chew and swallow. If swallowing solids becomes a problem, there can be a risk of choking. A person can be referred to specialists such as a Speech and Language Therapist (SALT) who will make a decision as to the type of foods that are desirable. If people have lost the ability to feed themselves, carers need to feed them. Carers in care homes must allow time for this process.

Loss of the use of arms – people with dementia may have forgotten what to do when they are asked or when it is suggested they participate in an activity. Carers may have to dress people such as by putting on underwear, and shoes, and even any jewellery or makeup and also have to comb a person's hair.

Caregivers will need to look after people's fingers in case they become stiff and curled in. Proper attention to fingernails can ease people's ability to undertake everyday activities, for example, a person may have difficulties with physical dexterity such as in holding items of cutlery. Carers need to ensure people's fingernails are not too long as they can scratch themselves or others.

Loss of the use of legs or poor mobility – people with dementia can forget how to walk or their joints may be stiff and painful. People may get cramps from sitting too long in one position, or are in pain on account of toenails needing attention. Carers will have to help people in all these circumstances. Carers need to check toenails, as with the fingernails, to ensure they are not causing pain when people are wearing shoes.

If walking along corridors, a caregiver should let people use the handrails. It may be a slow process for people to walk where they want to go, so carers must allow plenty of time. Some days, expedience may warrant the use of a wheelchair such as if there is an incontinence issue or walking has become hazardous.

> *It sounds like a lot of work but once you get in the habit of looking after all the areas of essential care, you and the team will find a working practice that serves people with dementia. A good working practice serves you and everyone else involved in care. In the end this will result in a fairly smooth running of the care home. It will be an exhausting, rewarding, and enjoyable job. What we are all looking for is best practice, for best care, all of the time.*

– A Tutor

Golden Rules

CARERS AT HOME can share personal experiences and learning with others by networking and by meeting with people through local carers' groups. Carers may make themselves aware of the condition of dementia via on-line sites. All the major care organisations and societies can be accessed on-line or via local authority information. Addresses and contact details can be found in phone books, libraries and doctors' surgeries.

CARERS ESPECIALLY IN CARE HOMES NEED TO regularly update their knowledge base of dementia care.

PEOPLE WITH DEMENTIA should receive respect at all times; they are experiencing terrible loss.

CHAPTER 6 — PHYSICAL HEALTH

"I've brought up two children, maintained a part-time job and combined this with being a housewife. I did school runs, joined clubs and a host of other activities people take on as part of adult life. I'm usually calm, good fun and fairly tolerant. So tell me why when I go to the care home to feed my mother I turn into a screaming (quietly!) demon! I play all the games she played with me to get me to eat when I was little. I played those same games with my children to get them to eat and it worked. So why will my mother not open her mouth and eat the food in front of her? It could take anything up to an hour to feed her and that may not include the pudding. I take my hat off to staff, I really do. I'm supposed to relieve staff so they can coax some other resistant eater. I am family, she should eat for me at least. The long and short of it is she's not wasting away, and I suppose as she's not active anymore her body needs less food but it does worry me."

– A Daughter

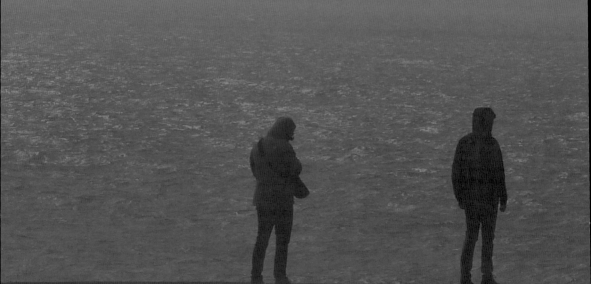

A-Z and reflections for carers

Appetite – caregivers will notice inconsistent eating habits in people with dementia. One day a person may eat huge amounts of anything including things off the floor like bits of string, bits of food, or food from someone else's plate. Another day the same person will neither drink nor eat no matter how meals are made tempting.

People can clamp their teeth or gums together and it may seem impossible to make any breakthrough in feeding them. Carers might have to call in a doctor to seek medical advice if it looks as if this attitude is going into its third day.

Ensuring that people eat and drink well is of primary concern whether they are in their own home, or in a care home, or other facility. The risk is high of malnourishment, dehydration and even starvation – leading to death, if all goes unchecked.

Also, if people wear dentures it may be necessary for carers to check they are in place and fit well. If people have their own teeth, carers need to ascertain there is no dental pain, no swallowing difficulty, or anything causing people to refuse food. It may just be people with dementia have forgotten what needs to be done in order to open their mouths, or they have not recognised the food or drink.

Bottom – the sacral region is where bed sores can start, which may be difficult to heal. This area of bed sores is usually at the base of the spine that becomes bony and protruding. Prevention is better than cure and a daily look at this area will keep carers aware of and ready for possible remedial action. Apart from a good diet and attention to skin care, particularly if the person is incontinent, changing people's position when they have been in bed for any length of time is essential. When people are awake but sitting for too long, encourage them to get up for a little walk every now and then to keep the circulation going. A moderate use of barrier cream after a wash is effective to prevent bed sores as well as the gentle patting of the area while the cream is being applied, to assist the circulation.

Diet – elderly and confused people tend not to eat large amounts, and usually go for easy carbohydrate food. Carers of people with dementia can offer small portions of nutritious food that is tasty and appropriate to their dental condition, any physical or medical constraints, and cultural preferences. Left to their own devices people with dementia may not eat all day yet claim they have had a big dinner.

Carers can tell as soon as they walk into a house whether a meal has been cooked recently such as by the smell or lack of food smells.

When people with dementia who have lived on their own end up having to be cared for in a care home, they can find the routine of regular food too much to cope with at first, they may lose their appetite initially and have to be fed.

> "A poor diet or one lacking in essential nutrients can result in anaemia, easy susceptibility to disease, dehydration, cramps, constipation, weight loss, tissue breakdown, mouth ulcers and a host of other related diseases. It's the considered opinion of many nutritionists and food experts that a diet containing all the essential components and possibly some supplements can be extremely beneficial in maintaining the physical and mental health of a person. Some carers seem to think that a meal heavily laced with carbohydrates offers a full and contented tummy – but in reality all it does is put weight on limbs already reduced in mobility and doesn't take into consideration the side effects of hypertension and obesity. An ageing person may still need a vitamin or mineral supplement to support a system that might be sluggish or poor at absorbing what little nutrients it is receiving. There are many ways of serving the meat and two veg option or pulses and vegetables if the person is vegetarian or if a person's dentition proves to be obstructive. Carers must ensure they see people eating their food."
>
> – A Nutritionist

> "It is my duty of care and responsibility to observe and record the mental and physical condition of patients and report back findings to the referrer such as a GP. On one occasion I visited and assessed the mental state of a single woman living on her own who once wandered into the surgery in an anxious state as she'd forgotten where she lived. On my visit, she appeared to be alert when she came to the door, let me in, and was quite chatty offering me a cup of tea that never got made although the offer was repeated several times. She was full of the things she got up to during the day and how she didn't need anyone to look after her as she was capable, after all she cooked for herself and went out on her own. I asked her what she'd cooked that day but she couldn't recall, just that it was delicious. I offered to make the tea for both of us and she allowed me into her kitchen. There were a lot of boxes of tea, and in the fridge there were numerous cartons of milk and packets of ham that hadn't been used or opened. There was no smell of food in the house, and my findings supported my suspicions she'd not cooked for days, maybe weeks, so she wouldn't have had hot meals. There were packets of opened biscuits. According to her neighbour, she did go out every day and came back with shopping. The contents of the cupboards and fridge revealed she was buying the same items over and over."
>
> – Community Psychiatric Nurse

Drinks – as drinking can also be a forgotten habit in the person with dementia, it is essential fluids are encouraged and offered and seen to be taken. There is a risk of dehydration, which can lead to confusion, mouth infections, urinary tract infections (UTI), sore throats, dry skin, constipation, and death. Some medicines can leave the mouth dry and with a bitter taste, so offering drinks regularly especially after giving tablets or liquid medication is crucial. Drinking habits will vary from day to day.

"*It's amazing how many residents in the care home can go from one day to the next with just sips of fluids. You can see them sitting with many drinks in front of them as everyone tries to tempt them with the various liquids, and they're not interested. They may take a sip or two to get you off their back but they don't seem to feel thirsty. On the other hand they may agree to take a drink, look as if they are going to drink it, then leave it.*"

– Care Home Worker

A sure sign of a drink left untouched is a build up of cups, mugs, feeders or other beakers all containing drinks. Carers need to take note of this non-drinking habit and report it rather than leave a drink nearby in the hope that recognition and thirst will cause people to succumb.

Ensure drinks are never hot enough to scald individuals, or the cup or glass is not so full that people's shaking hands spill the drink when they try to lift up the container.

"*Some feeder cups are fine until the drink is at the bottom – then when people, even if helped by a carer, try to drain the last drop they might squash their nose up against the lid, and they cannot breathe. In this situation, the choice is between drinking and breathing!*"

– Care Home Worker

Eyes – need attention to ensure they do not become sticky. Redness, puffiness, itchiness and weeping eyes can be irritating and interfere with a person's well-being. Eyes can become stuck down and infected. Some eye infections are contagious. Carers will need to report their observations to the GP or, if in a care home, to the person in charge.

Facial hair – if a female person with dementia needs shaving, and in her earlier life would not have wanted facial hair, then no matter what her age or condition the carer can try to do so. Shaving needs skill and care.

Footcare – as with most elderly people, feet do need to be looked after. Seek the assistance of a chiropodist or podiatrist if there are long nails, misshapen nails, ingrowing nails, bleeding and infected nails. A foot specialist will also observe the joints, the skin condition, any swelling or abnormalities, bunions and any corns or verrucas, which can be extremely painful. Extra care must be taken if the person is diabetic, due to poor circulation; healing to that area could be slow. Piercing or cutting the skin whilst attempting to trim people's nails could cause pain or infection.

Gentle foot massage, exercises to improve the circulation, and correct footwear are important. If a person is in a care home or admitted to one, the primary carer should ascertain arrangements regarding foot treatment such as if payment for this service is included in the fees.

Hearing – sometimes people with dementia are preoccupied, or only tuned in to particular voices, or cannot comprehend what is being said.

> **❝***Even if I do eventually end up almost shouting and the whole street can hear what I'm saying but dad can't hear, raising my voice doesn't always help, I have to find alternative ways of getting my message across.***❞**
>
> **– Family Member**

Vision – individuals with dementia may not perceive what others see no matter how people describe or show something. With all the changes going on in the brain, they may not be able to determine what they are looking at. They will not see colours properly or be able to distinguish between colours. When carers ask them to choose which outfit they would like to wear, they may not be able to recognise what they look at. Whatever the response, it is still best to involve and ask the person anyway.

People's perception of space and where objects are in a room will be different, for example, they may not realise a chair is not as close as they think, or not as high, or wide. They may reach for the chair, miss and then fall down or perch on the edge.

Carers might never be able to find out what an individual with dementia can see. Poor eyesight can encourage feelings of paranoia and hallucinations. Visual impairment may also be the reason why people and objects cannot be recognised, and why people lose interest in their food or their surroundings. Arrange to get people's eyes tested and encourage them to ensure they wear their glasses.

People's spectacles will get misplaced, so put them in a regular safe place and keep them clean or they will end up covered in food particles or dust and never worn.

Golden Rules

SERVE NUTRITIOUS MEALS and plenty of fluids little and often. Carers may get bored with the same meals but if these are the most liked then make the meal and give it. Large meals can sometimes put people off, and the food becomes wasted. Ensure people have eaten their food and taken plenty of fluids.

VISUAL PERCEPTION may make it difficult for people to see things as they are. Objects, people and places may be misinterpreted.

RESPOND EARLY to physical needs and infections, before they become problematic.

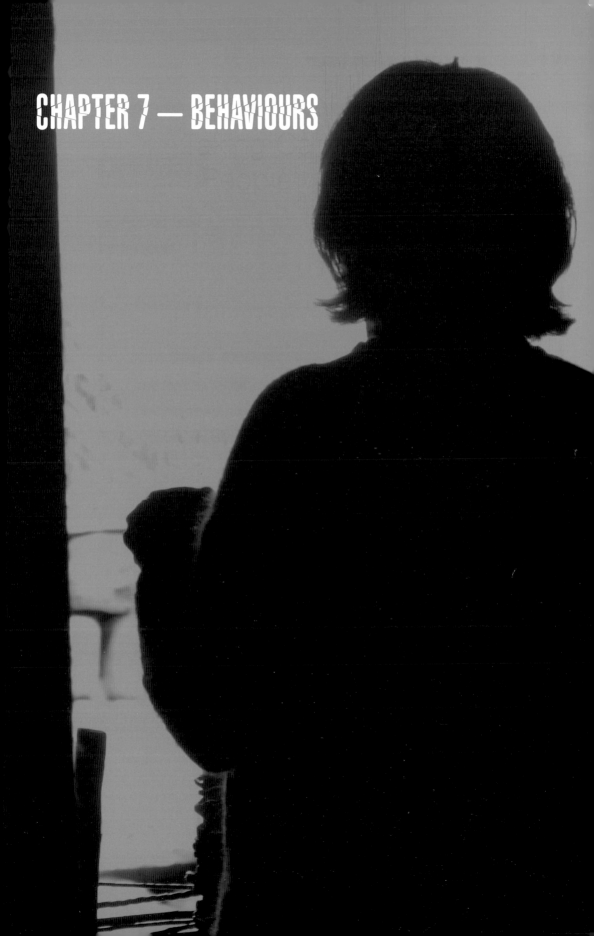

CHAPTER 7 — BEHAVIOURS

For a person with dementia all their behaviour has a purpose. Carers can try to find the root cause and motivation of people's behaviours, which is not always easy, but will assist understanding and caregiving.

A-Z and reflections for carers

Anxiety – occurs in dementia, sometimes showing with agitation and restlessness, which may be as a result of the way people feel on a particular day; they may be in pain, discomfort or disorientated. Agitated behaviours can be more noticeable in the evenings. Anxiety may also be present in carers as a nagging, persistent fear that things will get worse and they might not be able to cope.

Awareness – comes and goes in individuals with dementia. People may appear to be paying no attention or unaware. They may overhear things and repeat them. They may divulge family secrets much to the embarrassment of the family.

> ❝Today a friend came to visit and I did start complaining about how difficult father can be, when he calmly walked in to the kitchen, greeted us both, washed out his teacup and went out again.❞
>
> **– A Family Member**

Calling out – people with dementia may call out for no apparent reason. Another action is constant chatting to themselves or to anyone who is within earshot. What can be heard is a beautiful confused jumble of words from thoughts and whatever pops into the mind. They whisper words and sentences with inflexions and questions and look towards other people as if they should understand. They may start to cry when no-one responds, and carers may feel bad for not knowing what they are talking about.

> ❝When I hear someone calling out, I'll stop what I'm doing and run in quite a panic to see what's up. But if I ask them if they were calling, sometimes they might deny it or just not answer, having just suddenly been struck with silence.❞
>
> **– Support Worker**

Sometimes people will shout for help constantly and have no idea why, and they will not be able to explain what help they are shouting for when asked. People may call out for their husbands, or call the names of their children, and they can become distressed when the named person does not turn up. Residents in care homes might ask to go home, and they become upset when they realise it is not going to happen.

Visitors to a care home who may not be familiar with this behaviour have been known to approach staff to solicit help for a person they assume is distressed. Many attempts by staff to find the root of the calling for help can be necessary before the visitor realises the person is not in danger or discomfort.

On some days, people's conversation will be better than others and then carers could encourage the banter and exchange of comments, to help people enjoy the bits of memory that return, finding a fleeting involvement in what is going on. On bad days, it may be best for carers to pretend they know what people are talking about, to stay in the moment with them and enjoy whatever connection is possible.

Early morning waking – it may be that the person with dementia is incontinent and unable to carry on sleeping with a wet bottom. Another explanation may be that early risers have been put to bed early by carers who have done so in order for work, which could not be accomplished when people were awake, to be undertaken. Or it could be that people at home or in the care home had their meal early followed by bedtime at around 8pm. Next morning, at 6.30am, they would have gone twelve hours without food, their blood sugar level may have dropped, and they are lying awake disorientated trying to come round.

> *It's sometimes the case that a cup of sweet tea and a biscuit may be all that's needed to get people off to sleep again for another couple of hours.*

– **A Family Member**

Fighting – the cause of fighting may be fear, seclusion, confusion, ignorance. Some dementias cause people to fight carers every inch of the way the moment they or others lay hands on them. Even when carers say what they are going to do and have permission, people can still end up grabbing carers' hands or wrists tightly, causing pain and inaction. Carers may have been at the receiving end of fights, and injuries could be serious.

People are strong and their facial expressions can reveal they are serious about fighting. During a scuffle, it may be difficult for carers to be aware that people with dementia have no idea why and what they are doing. An activity such as putting on clothing or taking off a garment that is wet or soiled, or simply changing into day clothes or night clothes, can turn into a wrestling match – which carers will lose at times.

> *My daughters didn't believe me when I told them their dad throws away food I've cooked, and then asks me for it. They didn't believe me when I said he can spend up to two hours in the toilet with the door locked, and he'll not answer me. They didn't believe me when I said I was afraid of him as he looked mean and so angry when I asked him again what he was doing and that I wanted to use the toilet myself. I was becoming a nervous wreck with the daily battles and having to deal with my own illness unsupported by him. I was 77, having chemo at the time and was weak many days but still had to look after him. The thought of killing him or myself crossed my mind many times, but I never told my children, I told my friend. She was the one who suggested I tell my GP. One evening, one of my daughters came over as I had had a bad day following treatment. She asked where her father was; I said he was in the toilet. He was in there for at least all of the time she was there, and when he emerged, not realising she was with me, he started shouting at me for his tea. She realised then the truth of what I'd been saying all along. It was such a relief to be believed.*

– **A Wife**

Hugs – human contact can relieve tension and anxiety. Hugging can bring people close to each other.

Indifference – people with dementia may seem not to care what happens to them; they might reflect a lack of interest in everyday affairs, which is mirrored in their body language.

> " *My dad's behaving in the care home now exactly like he used to do at home, which drove me mad, and I expect it drives the staff mad, too. Sitting all day doing nothing except staring into space. Or staying in bed all day refusing to have a wash, refusing meals, or refusing to even answer us, wanting no contact whatsoever. I could have screamed.* "
>
> **– A Daughter**

Inertia – it may appear people with dementia have no energy or willingness to move or to do anything, or they may have forgotten what they could do. Inertia might mean people stare into space. Individuals may prefer just to sit quietly in their own world.

> " *Women in particular may spend the better part of their life working, looking after husbands, children, grandchildren, doing voluntary work, helping in their faith communities, being involved in charity work, and generally quite active. So when they're seen sitting staring vacantly into space in their own world – and enjoying, for once, their own thoughts without anyone making demands on them – it may be kinder to leave them alone. Of course, if a son or daughter feels their mother is apathetic and needs to be involved in activities to her benefit that's another matter but these can be overdone.* "
>
> **– Care Home Worker**

Injury – people with dementia are prone to fractures of the wrists, hips, legs, ankles. Caregivers may feel judged and guilty as if it is their fault when loved ones suffer injuries such as from a fall.

> " *One day a woman might walk across a floor she's traversed every day for practically eighty years, yet she trips over nothing, breaks something, and requires hospital attention. It's also easy for the skin to bruise if people are held too tightly or if they bump into furniture. Tight clothing like socks can impede circulation and it's not uncommon to see people sitting with their legs looking swollen above the level of the socks. People's feet and toes will then be cold and they may be experiencing pins and needles or even cramp but may be unable to let the carer know. When they try to stand up or get out of bed, they may fall.* "
>
> **– Care Staff Trainer**

Libido – even when some people with dementia are not seeking relationships, thoughts of sex may be in their mind. Carers should not be fooled into thinking people have forgotten the sexual act. Masturbation is not uncommon and the desire to have sex is not buried. Some cheeky flirtatiousness may be evident in people's speech and their actions such as when they grab their husbands, or wives, or carers or care staff, and then forget what the grabbing was about. Particularly, males with dementia are likely to find their intimate attentions unwelcome in care homes when their remarks and actions become embarrassing, or when they target vulnerable residents or younger care staff.

> "*I've heard many an elderly person say to a young nurse, 'Oh, If only I was 30 years younger.' And there are numerous times in care homes when one dementia resident climbs into another one's bed – and then has to be turfed out by staff, and the other person looks on perplexed.*"
>
> **– Care Home Worker**

> "*My mother had to be rescued by firemen when she forgot to turn off the oven and the smoke alarm went off in the warden-controlled flat. She was all over the firemen and had to be checked over by the female paramedic. When she was recounting the story, days later she claimed the firemen and the nurses had stayed behind and were having orgies in her bedroom.*"
>
> **– A Son**

Meddlesome – in care homes, people might go into someone else's room, look into their cupboards, get into their beds, or take items out of their room. Carers may have a struggle if they try to reclaim items from them to return to the owners.

> "*Some persons with dementia touch everything, including touching other people constantly and pulling at them and leading them away, or plucking at their clothes. They pick up stuff, put it down, pick it up, put it down, and pick up stuff belonging to other people, putting it usually where it may never be found – and they may never remember where they put things, and if they did they may not be able to tell us in a language we can understand. Around meddlers, the rule is: if people don't want stuff lost, don't leave it out.*"
>
> **– Care Home Staff**

Outings – for people with dementia, the procedure of going out can be fraught with difficulties and demands immense planning. Every move has to be taken into consideration such as should a person sit in the front or back seat in the car, or if it is necessary to take along a wheelchair.

Even a very short journey may have consequences. For example, if carers want to go quickly to a local shop, they question if they can leave a person with dementia in the house for five minutes. Carers will need to think about the problems that could occur in such situations. For example, when carers return after swiftly popping out for a few minutes, they could find a loved one lying in the home, suffering a fractured wrist, femur or ankle after a fall, or individuals may have been incontinent.

> ❝I decided to take my mother with me in the car to the corner shop, which was only a short journey. I wondered if I should leave her in the car while I nipped in, or should I take her in with me. I got to the shop and parked the car alongside so I could see her through the glass and vice versa. Telling my mother I wouldn't be long, I ran into the shop, grabbed a basket and hurriedly threw in items from the shelf, elbowed my way to the checkout and rushed back to the car. Mother was fast asleep; I needn't have worried or rushed.❞

– A Daughter

> ❝I took my mum to a superstore, but only to the supermarket section, and I planned when the shopping was over we'd go into the café for a cup of tea and a cake. As soon as I got mum out of the car I realised it would be a slow progress and wished I could put her in the front of the trolley the way my mum did me when I was a child. So we had to walk at a snail's pace along the aisles, and I let mum choose some items every now and then of her favourite foods. But mum decided not to like most of the foodstuffs she normally did yet I bought them anyway knowing they'd be eaten heartily in the week. Once or twice we almost lost each other when I moved further along the shelves in one direction to get something and mum, following her own instincts, moved in the opposite direction. What seemed like hours later we went through the checkout and into the café for the much-needed cup of tea. When we got up to leave there was a small puddle on mum's chair and her dress was clinging to her. So my message to other carers is to be prepared and think ahead. Although my mum didn't usually need a pad and I'd taken her to the toilet before we set off, we learnt that on occasions a pad was necessary to save us both from embarrassment.❞

– A Daughter

Spitting – some people with dementia have a habit of spitting, and it seems men are more likely to do so. Some will spit due to the taste medicines leave in their mouths, or the same medicine could encourage excess salivation. Sometimes food particles become trapped in people's teeth. When people have managed to work these particles free they spit them out. Others may spit for no apparent reason. It may be helpful to offer a drink after medication, or a rinse. If possible, get to the cause of the excessive salivation.

Swearing – people never known to swear during their lives may start swearing – and using offensive words and phrases – when they develop dementia. This practice is linked with anger and rage which they may not have expressed during their lives. Lack of inhibition can bring out the side of their nature that was repressed.

> ❝When I tell my friends about the way my husband carries on they can't believe me as on the few times they've seen him he's been as sweet as pie. I'm the only one who experiences the Jekyll and Hyde personality that is my spouse.❞

– A Wife

Toileting – carers can try to establish a good routine for people with dementia, which is influenced by individuals' consumption of food and drink. If planned well, the routine can save carers' time and energy.

> "I take dad to the toilet but I can't make him pee. Some time later I'll hear the sound of running water, and it's dad peeing up against a wall, or beside the wardrobe, outside the toilet door, in the plant pot, in fact anywhere he happens to be standing when he got the urge. There's the old trick of running the tap in the sink to encourage the flow of urine, but if I run it too hard I can't hear if he's doing a pee, or else I'll want to go myself but he can't be left alone!"

– A Son

> "I ask mum countless times if she wants to go to the toilet and she'll say no, but later on I might discover she's done her 'number one' exactly where she's sitting and I know nothing about it. Or I can spend at least 15-20 minutes in the toilet waiting for her to do one or the other but you can bet your life she may do neither in the toilet, she'll wait for some other place or some other time."

– A Daughter

Wakefulness – people might lie in bed whilst awake, causing no disturbance, or will quietly potter about in their own room. But some people awaken very early and then try to leave their own home or a care home. Carers need to keep the main door safely secured.

> "When my husband was at home, our bed routine was the same every night. We'd watch the news at ten, have a cup of tea and a biscuit; he'd check the doors; we'd go to bed and be asleep by eleven. Then he went in to a nursing home. As expected, he was unsettled, but apart from checking doors frequently he more or less stuck to the same routine we had at home. For no reason he started waking up at two and attempting to leave the home. When the carers asked where he was going, he'd say, 'To work.' Or, 'To the shop.' Or he wouldn't reply at all but would shake off the hand of anyone who tried to stop him. It didn't seem to matter it was pitch black outside, or raining, or he wasn't dressed properly, he was determined to get somewhere. My husband was a known walker and most of his day would be spent following staff around and being taken out in the garden for walks or joining in with activities. You'd think he'd be tired at night. Once, care staff put him back to bed eight times during the shift and that was after cups of warm chocolate, biscuits, toileting, handholding, gently soothing and leading back to bed, adjusting pillows or the bed; opening or closing windows, anything to persuade him his bed or his room was the most desirable place to be. Just when they thought they'd cracked it he'd be out of his bedroom again trying to leave. The staff positioned themselves halfway along the corridor so he could have a walk but go no further towards the exit. At other times he's tried to go into another resident's room and had to be stopped so that person's sleep was not disturbed."

– A Wife

Late night and early morning wakefulness and trying to leave the premises will be addressed in a care home where there is more than one member of staff and they can take turns to watch people. If the person is at home with one carer – who may be the same age and who needs sleep – then the situation can become difficult to control.

Walking – people with dementia seem to display many types of walking, which have diferent consequences. People might walk round in circles and have no idea where they are going, looking surprised when carers attempt to direct them. Or walking about can obstruct the way of a carer who is trying to do housework.

People with dementia might go upstairs and stop halfway as they forget their initial purpose, or restlessly pace from one room to the next, losing weight with the sheer calorie burn out.

When people are out with a carer, they may leave the safety of the pavement, or walk in the middle of the road. They may look purposeful when leaving a house, get lost, be unable to remember who they are, and carers have to call the police to find them.

Walking can mean they lose their way in a care home after using the en-suite toilet in their own room, then coming out and going into someone else's room to lie on a bed.

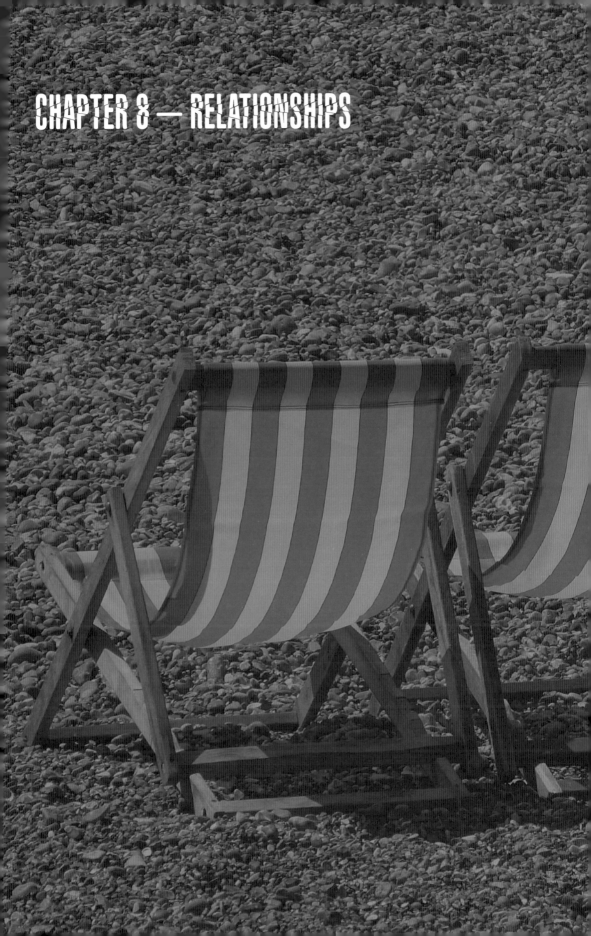

CHAPTER 8 — RELATIONSHIPS

When a person with dementia who needs a lot of attention comes to stay with other people such as a son or a daughter and family, some marriages or relationships may be tested and might not survive.

The energy and planning required to reorganise domestic arrangements and care for a person with dementia can sometimes take attention away from any disharmony that existed previously such as between a couple.

The move could give a shared goal between two partners preparing for the person to live in their home. Once it has been agreed that one partner's relative will move in to the family home, it can also mean the other partner will expect the same consideration with a relative who develops dementia.

If parents with dementia are to live in their children's homes, all the pros and cons of care must be examined, and the views of everyone taken into consideration. Also, the care of the person's pets will have to be reviewed, and decisions taken.

Brothers and sisters can become strangers, physically and emotionally, to the sibling who has taken in their mother or father. That lack of support can have a serious impact when it comes to caring for and coping with the parent who is experiencing dementia.

Lines of loyalty can be drawn up, and if the relative with dementia has had difficult relationships within the family then people might feel compelled to want other action. The decision to put the relative into a care home after only a short stay with them could be made very quickly.

Decisions about how to proceed with a parent who has dementia have caused rifts among siblings. Some might absolve themselves of responsibility and watch from a distance to see when and if the process of care goes wrong. Some brothers and sisters can remain close and helpful and are grateful for what is being done. Some remain close but unsupportive giving excuses about not being able to offer any help, or are full of unnecessary advice. Some siblings only criticise everything being done or push caregivers into making the decision to choose a care home for the parent – bringing guilt and shame to the carer.

> **"**I felt pressured into providing full-time care for my mother, while my brothers only looked after the finances. They rarely came over to see her or to find out how I was coping but were very quick to accuse me of overspending and playing the martyr.**"**
>
> – A Son

Golden Rules

CAREGIVERS COULD TRY if appropriate to involve other family members in the caring process, even if they never see them, such as by phoning or writing a letter to give a health update. Carers suggest it is advisable to delegate duties, have discussions on who will do what, and who will be the person to bring the family together for regular reports on expenditure. This support can relieve the burden on the main carer and share obligations and responsibilities among other people.

IF A CARE HOME IS THE BEST OPTION, there should be discussions on how the cost is to be met. Find out if the local council will part-fund the care; someone from an adult social care team, a social worker or the Citizens Advice Bureau (CAB) can give advice. It appears that local authorities may award costs differently.

Also, the main carer who has been living in the home of a parent may become homeless if the property has to be sold to pay for care home fees.

ELDERLY COUPLES might need to bring to their children's attention – or to inform other family members – that one or both of them increasingly requires more care.

SISTERS AND BROTHERS should be made aware of the distances people travel in order to visit a mother or father to provide care, and the sacrifices that are being made within their own families.

CARERS CAN SHARE their feelings or hurts such as with another person or in a support group, and discuss personal emotions and experiences. To withhold painful feelings can result in illness – and impact on the level of care that can be provided to dependents.

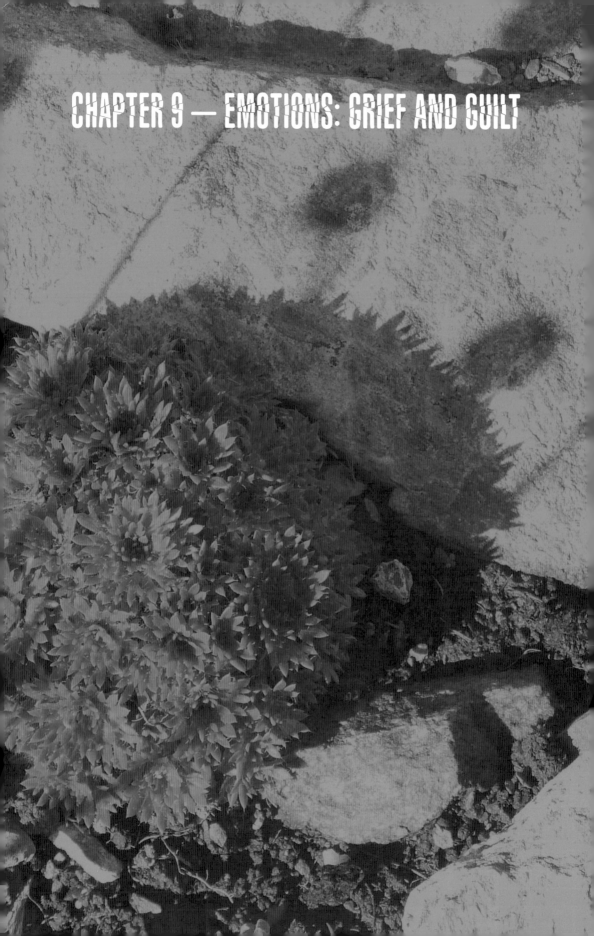

CHAPTER 9 — EMOTIONS: GRIEF AND GUILT

Grief is one of the most painful emotions felt by anyone involved in caring for a person with the onset of dementia leading into the full-blown illness. The grief can be for what is being lost and when carers become as strangers to the person with dementia.

People's loss of memory mean they do not know their loved ones and will never again recognise them as their spouse, or child, or sibling, or family members, no matter if family pictures are shown, or if children are brought to see them, or they are called mum or dad, or have memories suggested to them. The family loves them and can want to get into their brain to fix it – but then feel grief, as all know this is impossible.

On some days the individual with dementia will bear no resemblance to the person others have known. People may wonder about what has happened to their loved one whose soul lives inside the person they hardly recognise.

Family members may wonder if they will ever get their parent back, or their sibling, their child, their partner, and will rage against a mother nature that seems so cruel, or against the medical profession for not finding a cure. Grief of who they have lost to dementia will feel overwhelming at times.

Carers can seek out a support group or other ways to express their feelings of grief and try to process their emotions for recognition and healing.

Guilt is a painful emotion that can set in when people reflect on their dependent relative and memories come to their mind. If caregivers keep their job and go to work part time, they might feel guilty for the relief of leaving the house – their only time off away from the demands on them. Or carers can feel guilty for living so far away and unable to do anything, or guilty about having to choose between caring for a husband with dementia or letting the family find a care home for him.

People feel guilty when, aware a loved one with dementia will not know if they visit, they stay away from the care home. Or people can feel guilty about the fact their guilt is a secret and they wonder what others would think about them. People may look as if they can manage everything, but to themselves they might feel a terrible guilt inside.

> **❝**I feel guilty because I asked myself how I could feel so resentful at having to look after this person after all she's been to me. Why do I feel like running away and letting someone else have the hassle? I began to be guilty for feeling hard done by even though at the time it was recognised, and I agreed, that I was the only one without ties so there was nothing really to prevent me from looking after mum and dad. There were all the ifs: if the others didn't have husbands, wives, children, commitments, jobs they couldn't possibly leave; if they didn't live so far away, then of course they would do it or be down like a shot, to give me a break. I only have to ask. But, I blame myself. For who was it who said no when the nursing home was mentioned? Me. Now, I feel guilty because in my tiredness I call her names when she's being so exasperating and stupid. I feel like slapping her when she has been incontinent of pee or pooh or both and then takes a delight in playing with them and leaving streaky marks on the walls and bits of it wherever she has touched. Most things can be stomached but that seems worst of all, and I may have been rougher than intended in my anger.**❞**

– A Daughter

> ❝I feel guilty because I feel hemmed in and trapped, I seem to have lost my freedom, I have no life. I can't even take a good holiday without first having to plan everything down to the last detail in case something goes wrong while I'm away. In my more maudlin moments especially if I've finished off the day with a glass of wine, I ask myself when did I last go to the cinema, out for a meal. I imagine everyone else is having a good time except me, and because I am too proud to ask for help or to admit that it is all too much now, no one knows what I feel or how I feel.❞

– A Son

> ❝When I do go out I have no conversation, I'm preoccupied thinking my mobile is going to go off any minute and the sitter will want me to go back home. Most of my conversation these days is about her routine and I try to think up exciting ways with steamed fish and prunes. I tell myself I should be a devoted caring child; after all, she did as much for me and made sacrifices for me when I was growing up. She went without so I could have some things and it is only right that I should do as much for her now that she's in need. But I am so tired. Who is looking after me or looking out for me? I feel old, unloved and undesirable.❞

– A Daughter

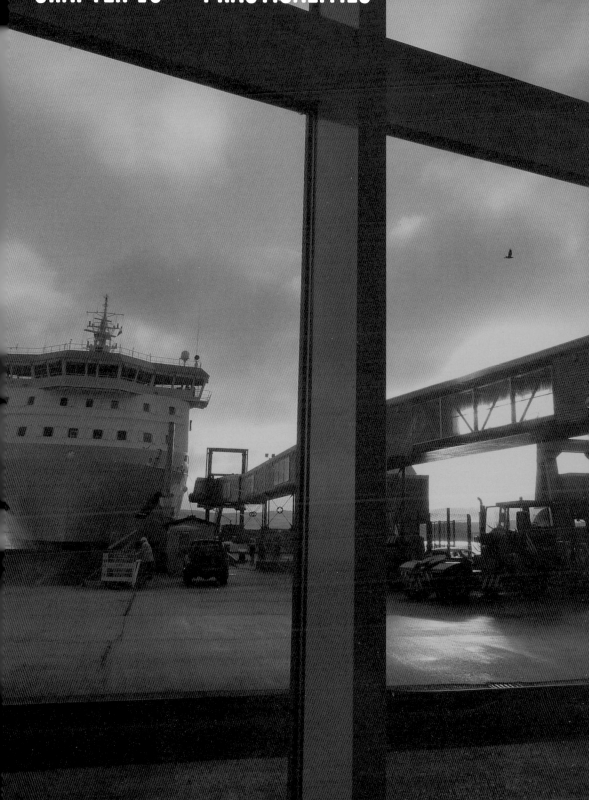

CHAPTER 10 — PRACTICALITIES

A-Z and reflections for carers

Allowances – primary carers who are providing care for at least 35 hours a week may be entitled to Carer's Allowance. The person being cared for may also be eligible for an Attendance Allowance and other benefits. These allowances and benefits can be worth pursuing to help with bills and other demands on finances.

It can be useful to obtain the advice of others who have already been through the claims application process as they could make the task much easier of filling out the lengthy and sometimes complicated forms.

Organisations such as the Citizens Advice Bureau (CAB), Age UK, the Alzheimer's Society, the Department of Work and Pensions (DWP), Carers UK, and Care for the Carers will be useful in guiding people through the maze of literature. The forms may be available in different languages.

Commode – an essential toileting aid, it can be disguised to look like living room furniture. Convenient for carers if it is positioned near the bed and after use will need to be emptied. It can also become a tripping hazard if not positioned carefully – and if not used can become a hiding place for various objects.

Daycare – a service that can relieve the burden of care on primary caregivers. It can give carers a short respite break. Find out from the local council how to access daycare services; inquire about transport arrangements and how often daycare can be provided.

Hearing aid – people can need a hearing aid but it can be uncomfortable and fiddly so it may not be worn by the person; it might not be in the correct ear; it can whistle like a kettle; even when it is turned up to its full extent people may still have to shout. Although a hearing aid is initially fitted by a specialist, carers might notice some time after that it does not fit as snugly and has to be adjusted. Or perhaps later it will be found left unused in its box complete with the spare set of batteries, or down the side of a chair, or is never found at all.

Incontinence underwear – readily available on the market. Some products are disposable, some are washable, and although many are for the wearers, there are other products that can protect bed linen or furniture.

There is padded underwear that comes already made up that people can slip on like an ordinary pair of pants, with a colour strip which lets carers know when pants have been soiled by the wearer. Some products called nets secure a pad in place.

Padded underwear is particularly useful at night when the daytime toilet routine would have stopped but the person continues to pass urine. Copius amounts may be passed during the night by a bladder whose ability to hold volumes would have been under-estimated.

Ordinary underwear can hold on to stains and lose its elasticity especially around the waist on account of the numerous washings.

" *There is one drawback with light-coloured underwear. Who wants to spend all day washing these items so the brown stains to the back do not embarrass you when they are hung out to dry? I took turns to look after my aunt and felt personally to blame when I couldn't shift the streaks. I felt as if I'd be judged and found to be neglectful.* "

– A Niece

Some suppliers may deliver protective pads and sheets to the household. It is worth reaching friendly terms with suppliers for times of emergency.

Money – caring and making life comfortable for a person with dementia can be expensive. Family carers may have to sell their parents' home or remortgage their own depending on where people end up living such as in a care home. Whether the carer receives state assistance or any kind of benefit, care provision is a significant expense.

Money can become an issue among family members. The primary carer may be accused of mismanaging a parent's money or of not exercising prudence. People may not be aware of the prices for care staff such as live-in staff or personal assistants.

Nightwear – can be practical; invest in a variety. Some nightdresses are fastened with velcro from shoulder to hem or with a discreet crossover opening at mid back to allow easy access to the toilet. There are short-sleeved and long-sleeved versions but think carefully before using the long-sleeved version as people may have powerful elbows and dressing could prove difficult.

" *A full length, long-sleeved nightdress with three or four cute little buttons at the neck and wrist, topped off with a lace trim at collar and cuff has been known to turn well-experienced, fully-trained staff almost into maniacs when faced with having to undress the person with dementia in one of their fighting moods in the middle of the night after they have their first bout of faecal incontinence.* "

– Care Home Worker

Pyjamas are popular with both males and females but are not always practical if carers have to keep taking them off when they are soiled or wet. Loose nightshirts and padded underpants seem to be a better idea.

Bed socks are ideal for cold feet; most elderly people suffer with poor circulation and may not get off to sleep if their feet feel like blocks of ice.

Mittens are worn by those who have a tendency to scratch their skin as the bed or room gets warm, or they have a skin condition.

Slippers – there are a number of styles on the market in a range of patterns and designs. The most popular is the slipper with velcro strap, adjustable for all types of feet including ones with bunions. It can be useful to buy many pairs, and they are usually washable and quick drying.

Stockings – can be adjusted above the knees or mid thigh, without making a tourniquet of them at the top. Another advantage of the stocking is that it will be easier for carers to change damp or soiled underwear – just remove the offending garments and replace. But if a person is wearing tights, these become wet and soiled along with everything else and have to be rolled down with the contents, while the carer tries to prevent the offending matter from making a bad situation worse.

> ❝To put tights on an unyielding, cross-legged, sometimes fighting, woman requires a skill that cannot be taught. When tights aren't properly adjusted the wearer can be seen walking like a robot or like a baby with a nappy because the gusset hasn't reached the groin and is somewhere mid-thigh between crotch and knees. No such problem with stockings.❞
>
> **– Care Worker**

If carers buy several pairs of stockings in the same colour then these can always be matched up when one of them needs discarding. This common-sense advice can be especially helpful for husbands or children looking after a spouse or a parent single-handedly.

Underwear – for general use includes bras, vests, half slips, underpants, knickers, stockings and socks. Carers can make sure of a plentiful supply to give choice.

Urinals for men – portable containers for males to urinate in. Some are made from washable, durable, hard plastic and some from recycled cardboard and can be thrown away. Urinals have a tendency to fall over especially when full, or to conceal urine in the base. Unless carers are diligent, they will only be aware there is stale urine in the container by the smell pervading the room.

> ❝It can be quite a problem trying to get the male organ into the urinal; its size, floppiness, and ability to extend itself to be placed into the opening of the urinal is greatly reduced by age and complicated by the confusion. It's better to learn how to handle that part of his anatomy and get the urine into the container, because the merits of contained urine far outweigh the demerits of wet clothing and bedding.❞
>
> **– A Carer**

Wills – keep the Will updated to avoid it being contested. People who are relatives of the deceased are not automatically entitled to anything in the person's Will. In care establishments, no member of staff is allowed to witness the signing of a Will or to benefit from a resident's estate. If a person wants to leave something such as a garden seat to the care home then that bequest is usually acceptable. A **Living Will** specifies decisions people would like to be made on their behalf in the event of them becoming incapable of making or communicating a decision. See also **Lasting Power of Attorney** in Chapter 15.

> *It was good to have a Living Will for my mother and prevented a lot of end of life panicking. Mum together with the other children and our solicitor helped to draw up what was called a directive, which proved extremely useful when she developed severe bronchitis in her 90s and had been suffering with Alzheimer's since her 60s. She had stated that she would not want her life prolonged including by the use of antibiotics. Her GP signed a form called a Do Not Attempt Resuscitation (DNAR) and everyone knew about it. It doesn't stop you from feeling that you're letting your mother die, but because we knew her wishes and we were all together when the end was near, it felt good her wish was granted. We didn't want to see her suffer, and she wouldn't have wanted that herself, either.*

– A Daughter

Zimmer frame – a handy piece of equipment when people need a walking aid and have been measured up for their own frame. But even when people have been fitted for their individual frame, they may refuse to use it. In a care home they might find one that belongs to someone else, which will be too short, too high, with wheels or without, and difficult or awkward to handle. It will be abandoned in a corner with many other walking aids, alongside wheelchairs. The independence people have been encouraged to achieve is then lost.

> *Some people become well versed in the art of walking with the Zimmer, but other people can be seen carrying it a few inches off the floor while they shuffle along, and in one case a woman was seen carrying hers over her head!*

– Care Home Worker

Golden Rules

DO NOT skimp on the provision of incontinence underwear and pads. They can be expensive but they are worth the cost.

DO NOT purchase fussy night clothing such as nightdresses with numerous buttons and bows as it can hamper the caring process.

DO NOT forget to involve the family in legal matters. Through a solicitor people can prepare a Lasting Power of Attorney (LPA) covering health and welfare, and finances. It can also be best to employ the services of a solicitor to draw up a Will. Check if a Living Will has to be drawn up.

INFORM all or at least one other family member that the LPAs and the Will are being prepared, and where they are filed.

IF POSSIBLE, PREPARE the LPAs and the Will before people with dementia deteriorate in mental faculties and physical health. Otherwise family members could legally challenge decisions, contest the Will, causing lasting bitterness as well as distress and expense.

DO KEEP all documentation, including bills and bank statements, in one place. It is advisable for family members to be made aware of where these documents are stored.

CHAPTER 11 — CARING AT HOME

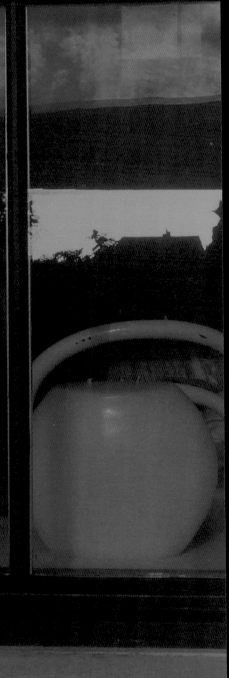

"My dad's marvellous. He's not as able as he was, and he's five years younger than my mum who's 86. She's on her way to dementia and has been slowly going that way for the past three to four years. She can't go out on her own; he won't let her go out on her own. We've banned him from driving her about, but luckily where they live he can walk to the shops; everyone knows them. She tells him what she wants (from the shops) and he goes out to get it. Between them they muddle through; they seem content. My fear is one of them will deteriorate and take the other with them. He enjoys looking after mum and rarely complains."

– A Daughter

The term primary carer is used for a person who has the most responsibility in looking after an individual with dementia who resides at home or in the carer's home.

Carers are advised to declare to local authorities and others they are the main caregiver, in the event of something happening that takes them away from the person receiving their care.

All carers carry a weight of responsibility, and caring is often an unpaid arrangement with people giving up jobs, education and relationships in order to look after the person diagnosed with dementia.

A carer is also someone who looks after another person for long periods of time. Sometimes people think they only do what another would do in their circumstances such as look after a wife or a husband or a partner. It might seem as if caring is automatically down to the spouse or the partner as an inevitable part of the relationship.

But to become a carer is to accept a specific role and way of life. Spouses and partners who become the carer of someone with dementia can find pressures emerge due to the different type of relationship.

Associations for carers recognise the stresses involved when people have to look after someone who is chronically ill. A carer's role can include dealing and coping with a person's incontinence, restlessness, wakefulness, aggression, and a host of other issues. When carers are the older spouse or partner they may have to deal with their own vulnerabilities, or carers may have health problems or emotional pain.

A charity such as Care for the Carers in East Sussex runs groups and forums that give a welcome platform enabling carers to discuss their problems openly and not feel so overwhelmed by their duties; to have respite breaks; to share experiences and advice on their emotional and physical well being, and to be recognised as individuals in their own right.

Forums and groups allow caregivers to be heard and have their feelings closely listened to and taken into consideration.This support can help carers use information divulged in groups to improve their own way of life and if possible the life of the person they are looking after. Resource materials, information, and advice regarding finances, form-filling and access to community groups are among the many ways that caregivers' needs are acknowledged.

Caregivers can discover strategies they could employ for themselves to reduce the effects of stress and address the demands of giving constant attention to the person with dementia.

A-Z and reflections for carers

Able – the initial question primary carers need to ask themselves about long-term care or short-term care is whether they are able and willing to do the caring. It may seem that they will be expected to do everything.

Caregivers need mental strength, physical stamina and to be in charge of their own faculties. Carers need their senses in good working order – and an extra one like having eyes in the back of the head! They need excellent dexterity and to be quick on their feet; to be able to go with very little sleep for days on end.

Carers need to be able to stay calm and not escalate a situation such as when accused of something by the person with dementia they know is untrue – and it seems as if a different truth could be beaten out of them.

Carers need to be able to hear swear words that are unfamiliar and shocking coming from a person who never swore – and to not be embarrassed if other people come in to the home when the swearing is taking place.

Caregivers need to be almost telepathic on some days as the person with dementia might refuse to speak and not answer even basic questions. They can develop non-verbal skills to communicate with and be understood by the one receiving their care.

Carers also require the ability to make sense of difficult to understand words or phrases, jumbled words, and to read people's body language that conveys needs such as the necessity to use a toilet urgently. They need to find ways to comprehend people's behaviour, for example, a person may just be angry or crying for a reason that is not apparent at the time to the caregiver.

Accusations – as well as theft, caregivers may be accused of intrusive actions. People with dementia become good at blaming others and making charges about them, particularly in the early stages of the illness. Children, partners or other carers may be accused of stealing money, or the pension book, or jewellery, or anything that cannot be found by the person making the allegation.

People with dementia can be so convincing caregivers might be sucked in and start thinking to themselves that theft could be possible by the person being accused.

A spouse or a partner who is known by everyone to never go out can be accused of having affairs, or of never being at home. In reality, a person may be afraid to go out in case their loved one with dementia would do something damaging in their absence.

> ❝Dad would be sitting in the same room as my mum, and when I rang up to find how things were and asked after my dad, the reply from mum was, 'He's not here, he's out with his girlfriend!'❞
>
> – A Daughter

Activity – during the early years of dementia it is possible to enjoy a fairly active life with a loved one. If people diagnosed with dementia are still capable of living on their own, they can continue doing what they are accustomed to; carers can keep alert from a distance. When assistance is needed for tasks that are becoming problematic the primary carer can step in.

A carer's main concern will be to preserve a quality of life that is going to change. There may be fun, sadness, enjoyment and exhaustion. Carers are encouraged to pursue a holistic lifestyle for their loved one, encompassing mind, body and soul.

While people with dementia are still able to self-care they can attend clubs and groups that can keep them mentally and physically active. In the home, carers will need to find their own way to avoid boredom from setting in although sometimes that can be a frustrating task.

> *Mum liked to knit, and bags of multi-coloured wool with knitting needles were provided by the care home when she went in for respite care. At home mum will sit for days on end with the wool on her lap, and if we are not careful it will end up stuffed down the side of her chair, or with food bits all over it when she refuses to relinquish it during meal times.*

– A Daughter

Arms – one outcome of dementia eventually is a loss of ability for self-care. Primary caregivers may have to help the person get dressed every time. However, it can be in the person's best interest to help in the act of dressing so the activity of taking physical care is not forgotten.

Apathy – some people with dementia appear to have a lack of interest in everything around them.

> *I was nearly reduced to tears when I couldn't get a response from my husband for a couple of days in a row. He sat there like a sack, eyes unfocused, no expression on his face, and barely opening his mouth to eat or drink – as if he'd already given up. No matter what I tried to coax him with, he showed no interest. I was becoming frustrated and tired with all the effort I alone seemed to be making.*

– A Wife

Armchairs – can seem to be lovely pieces of furniture in which the person is content to sit for days on end, either sleeping or staring. It can be wise to place a protective pad or sheet on the chair before a person sits down, in case of accidents. Armchairs can reek of bodily smells and carers may find themselves regularly cleaning to rid rooms of the odour.

Awake – can be how the caregiver and care-receiver spend some nights. The person with dementia might sleep all day, or parts of the day; carers would have been busy all day attending to personal and household needs. At night, a carer may be too tired to sleep – and resort to a 'help' such as alcohol to cope with circumstances. Many home carers reflect how they feel guilty using this crutch to help them get through the nights.

Backache – comes in carers from fetching and carrying, pulling and tugging, bending and straightening. From bending to make beds that are low to lifting mattresses that are heavy. From going to and fro; from walking up and down stairs. There is a high incidence of backache among nursing staff, care staff, and home caregivers. Apart from providing for the physical care of a person with dementia, practical demands include laundry, shopping, bed-making, cooking, cleaning. In a care home, staff do these individual tasks – but caregivers in a family home can have all the responsibility put on them.

Bathing – caregivers living at home may not need to bathe the people they care for every day. Vital body oils can be lost by too much washing and soaping, which may lead to scaly dry patches on areas of skin.

If carers do not have proper support, and unless they are fit and strong, then bathing an individual one-to-one in the bathroom should be avoided except perhaps if the person with dementia is fairly lightweight, agile, and comprehending of a carer's intention. Even in care homes it is advisable to have two staff present during the process. Sometimes a hoist or sling is needed when compliance is not forthcoming. For a primary caregiver at home it can be far more difficult to lift the person into or out of a bath.

It is important to assemble everything needed beforehand, or to only bathe the person when extra help is available. There are risks in leaving an elderly person in the bath. If additional help in the home is unavailable, a daily wash can suffice.

At home, the activity of bathing can be fraught with danger even if there is a slip mat in the bath, a bath stool or support rails. A slippery floor can be an added risk. Before any aids are considered or fitted it can be advisable to consult with an occupational therapist. Fitments will be adapted and adjusted to suit individual need.

There are a wide range of baths and showers available; these can be expensive. Some people use a plastic chair in the shower cubicle, or have a seat fitted under the shower, or put in a wet room or other type of shower, if there is space and money to convert an existing bathroom.

> **"***I told my wife what I intended to do and took her bath things into the bathroom first. I got her into the bath without too much trouble and washed all that needed to be washed, or that I could reach; she didn't help at all. Things started to go wrong when I attempted to get her out of the bath. She seemed to have lost interest and did not want to get out and appeared to forget where she was. I had already pulled the plug to let some water out in anticipation of getting her out, and her skin was damp and slippery. I kept talking to her all the while, calling her by name and telling her what I was going to do. I tried to heave her under the armpits but she became heavier and heavier, and with the bath slippery on all sides she was getting frightened and started shouting and hitting me. I don't know how many towels I put on top of her to keep her warm as she was now lying full length in the bath and refusing to help. In the end by sheer determination and brute energy only frustration can give you, I managed to get her two legs to hang over the side of the bath, and with one of my legs in the bath I somehow heaved the rest of her onto the chair I'd placed alongside. It took all my energy and strength to finally get her sorted, I vowed never again. I'm 80, what would've happened to her or to me if as a result I had a heart attack?***"**
>
> **– A Husband**

Bed – may present a problem if a carer is faced with a sometimes helpless individual. As with any mechanical aid, beds might not always function. On good days – when a carer feels strong and able for anything – the bed on wheels is a real asset. On bad days – maybe when a carer feels worn out – the bed can behave like a supermarket trolley moving heavily in one direction or in a contrary fashion. A divan bed with no wheels at all can be heavy and cumbersome to move.

Bed making – the bed has to be made. If too many sheets or blankets are put on the bed, they may all become soaked with urine. If too few blankets are put on the bed, the person with dementia may complain of being cold, which can be difficult for carers to hear especially at a time when they might have fallen asleep at last.

The ideally-made bed seems to be: mattress protector; fitted bottom sheet; pad or protector to protect those sheets; a flat top sheet; a couple of blankets or a duvet. The number of pillows used depends on personal preference or the way a person wants to be positioned in bed for greatest comfort.

In a care home or hospital, beds are made with two people working in unison and with all bedding readily available. At home, carers have to consider their own capabilities and the efficiency of washing and drying facilities.

Bedpan – caregivers may have to help a person to use a bedpan. To place a bedpan well and remove it successfully is a difficult task plus there can be unforeseen problems.

The person with dementia might indicate they want to pee but when bedpans are removed it is obvious something else has been deposited there – and carers would not have been asked for paper. Carers should keep a roll of toilet paper handy by the bedside.

Carers also have to be adept at removing the bedpan with one hand and keeping the person on their side with the other hand – so the individual does not roll over and soil the bed whilst the carer tries to clean them up. During this time, the person, having forgotten what is going on, may be struggling to lie back on the bed.

People may be heavy and carers can start to feel their wrists and arms becoming painful in the process of helping someone use a bedpan. The activity ideally needs another person to help but if carers are unsupported, they have to find their own technique.

Clothing – can pose a problem especially when carers are trying to dress someone. Clothing must be easy to remove without causing exposure. Also, to clothe someone takes a while, which can put extra demands of time on carers.

Clothing should be worn as near as possible in the style to which the person has been accustomed. It should be appropriate to both indoors and outdoors – depending on the weather. Clothing can be added to if the person is going out. If there are draughts in the home or the person is known to be always cold, extra socks or a scarf can be worn indoors.

People may have been smart dressers before dementia and that habit can still continue. It is possible to dress stylishly with elasticated trousers, jeans or leggings, with smart bright jumpers, cardigans and tee-shirts, and dressy shoes or slippers with velcro strapping.

Stockings, knee highs or loose fitting unelasticated socks can keep the feet warm and can prevent restrictions in the calf area that may interfere with the circulation. Choose shoes and bedroom slippers that can be easily and quickly removed. Sports bras seem to be less restrictive and fiddly than bras with hooks and eyes. Poor laundry care can cause items to shrink.

> ❝*The last thing I want is to change a full set of clothing three or four times a day because I put on to mother a pair of tights that she is unable to fathom when she goes to the toilet.*❞
>
> **– A Daughter**

Confusion – people with dementia can become slower and muddled and may start a job but not complete it on account of the shortened attention span, or forget what they were meant to be doing and how to do it. Observations in one type of dementia show that recognition of familiar objects is lost, or that familiar objects can appear to be something else. Trying to speak for the person or to guess what they want to say may not always help, as the introduction of too many suggestions could cause further confusion.

Constipation – carers have to address this issue in a person with dementia. Some elderly people will have used aperients and laxatives to move their food along and would have been raised on a routine of having 'to go' every day, if possible after breakfast. At this stage of their lives, when they are no longer engaged in much activity, and peristalsis is slowed down, the body seems to hold on to anything it has eaten – unless forced out by self or medical treatments. Constipation has been known to cause confusion, distress, discomfort and irritability.

Dentures – carers will have to deal with a person's top set, bottom set, or full set. Some fit, some do not, and may not be worn when most needed such as at mealtimes, and they are easily misplaced. Never leave dentures lying about and out of their pots because people can move them and they may be lost.

Dentures need daily attention with toothbrush, toothpaste, or cleansing tablets, or even a quick rinse after each meal so bits of food do not remain stuck in the gums. Preferably, carers should remove the denture fix each time so there is not a build up of it leading to a bad fit and causing a sore mouth.

Carers should never put their fingers into a person's mouth to remove teeth unless the individual has been told or shown what the carer intends to do. Teeth in a confused person's mouth can give a very nasty bite.

Carers should never place a toothbrush into a person's mouth unless the individual has been told or shown what the carer intends to do. Dentures or even people's own teeth can clamp down on toothbrush handles. The carer would have to spend much time trying to dislodge the toothbrush without causing damage to the person's mouth.

Carers should never give an antiseptic mouthwash and expect the person to rinse, gargle and spit out – the person may swallow it.

Despair – an emotion felt by many relatives and carers when nothing seems to work; there is a real danger of giving up on the person for whom they are caring.

Diarrhoea – can be part of an infective process. If diarrhoea is infective – and carers may know this by the smell, the frequency, and the amount of liquid motions passed – then it would be wise to call in the GP as the issue can be serious. Infective diarrhoea is contagious, best dealt with in isolation and treated immediately.

Care homes may have policies in place on the treatment of infectious diseases – and include seclusion and isolation as part of the treatment. In a person's own home, caregivers have to be careful and let the GP know if the diarrhoea remains loose and liquid as there could be a risk of dehydration.

Embarrassment – some carers find the intimacy of providing care can be awkward and embarrassing. Some men express they have no real idea of what to do when it comes to giving mum or dad a wash or a bath. Both men and women have probably never seen their parents' private parts. The intimacy that personal care calls for reduces many people to tears. The parental role of caring has been reversed.

> *I want to reassure newcomers to care that the bathing and toileting routine becomes a little easier once they have done it a few times. We can feel we want to give a loved one their privacy and so try not to hover in the doorway of the toilet when they've gone in to use it. But we know that if we don't stay close, all manner of things can happen. Our loved one may end up playing with the pooh or pee because they've forgotten what they're meant to be doing. They're also likely to get up from the seat before they've finished so have an 'accident' on the floor. If they attempt to clean themselves it would be with just one or two squares of toilet paper, which they have painstakingly and neatly torn off from the roll.*
>
> **– A Family Carer**

Embarrassment can also occur when carers assist people with the toilet routine. If some people with dementia are left to their own devices in the toilet, problems that can occur include putting soap or the whole toilet roll down the toilet bowl, or washing their hands in very hot water. If people have attempted unsuccessfully to wash their hands there can be bits of the brown stuff all over tap heads, the walls, the towels, and everywhere. To avoid the worst of outcomes, carers might need to go in to the toilet with people and to look away, respectfully waiting to deal with difficulties if necessary.

> *My mum became unable to care properly for herself when she was in her late 80s. Prior to that she had been diagnosed with Alzheimer's but managed alright. I would phone her every day and as I didn't live too far away, I'd drop in about two to three times a week to see how she was getting on. We'd watch a bit of television, and I'd make sure she got into bed before I locked her in. That arrangement worked for some time until my sister mentioned she noticed mum wasn't changing her clothes as often as before, and did I notice anything? I didn't really. The crux of the matter came when my sister was going on holiday and said she'd been making sure that mum washed and changed her clothes more regularly, and I'd have to do it while she was away otherwise we'd have to arrange for someone to come in. I still didn't realise what was really involved. My sister wrote out the routine that was to be followed for bathing or washing mum. On paper I thought it was easy enough. I decided I'd not bathe my mum as I'd never seen her naked and knew I'd be more embarrassed than her, so it was to be a wash. Mum said she needed the toilet so I sat her on it and told her to call me when she was finished. When she didn't call after a good while I glanced in to see what*

was happening; she was sitting there looking bewildered with toilet paper in her hand. I said, 'Clean yourself up mum. And we'll have a nice wash.' Nothing. I said, 'Mum, you need to wipe yourself before we have that wash.' Still nothing. I was horrified at what dawned on me. I'd have to wipe her bum and wash her private parts. To cut a long story short, I got her to stand up while she held on to the sink, tried to wipe her rear end – with my face averted – which only led to her peeing on my hand; nothing caught in the toilet paper. When I tried to wash her private area, I couldn't see but hoped I was reaching the parts that needed to be cleaned. All the while my mum stood in silence, and I got the job done. I was knackered. 'All done mum.' And she said, 'You are a good boy.' I burst into tears. After that I can't say it got any easier but I preferred my sister to do the bathing and washing."

– A Son

Faecal incontinence – carers may have to deal with faecal incontinence in the person with dementia. The caregiver may be alerted by a persistent lingering smell wafting when a person passes by. Sometimes loose motions will happen near the toilet but also in a place where the person has been walking, so then it will be carried around everywhere. If the person has an awareness that what has been done needs cleaning up, this can present another problem as attempts to help can make a bad situation worse.

If people have been wearing incontinence pads or pull ups, carers might be able to remove these, then wash and clean people up, and put on clean pads. Without them, stuff will seep out and stain whatever people have been sitting on; the person with dementia will then require a bath. Sometimes no matter what carers do, the smell lingers in a room and throughout the house. There may be a need for air fresheners, and special cleaning products for rooms and fabrics.

"*My wife turned on me one day all of a sudden, as if I was harming her or something. I'd just spent the better part of half an hour cleaning her up without any help from her, and maybe I was a bit harsh. I'm sorry to say she looked ugly, and her behaviour was ugly. I couldn't think of her in a nice way after that and it made me feel guilty.*"

– A Husband

Faeces – people with dementia may have a fascination with the faeces and will remove this from their bottom, their bed, or their pads, and spread or smear it everywhere perhaps in a misguided attempt to get rid of it. If noticed early, then the person may be cleaned up quickly and things can go back to normal. If the incident is only found after being alerted by smells and the sight of excrement in places, it may involve a lot of work to clean the person's hands, nails, and any other part of their body involved. Then comes the painstaking work of removing it also from the walls, door handles and other places. Some carers at home have admitted this behaviour can make them feel disgusted.

Falling – falls can happen often and apparently for no reason. People may fall over on a plain flat surface which is familiar to them, and they will sustain bruises and injuries that can make caregivers seem like an abuser or neglectful. In some types of dementia, repeated falling is common.

People with dementia may forget their balance is upset or that they have had a stroke. While they may want to be mobile, in reality they are not as capable as they feel. People also fall out of bed; they roll out and cannot stop themselves – or they make no attempt to clutch on to something when they feel themselves falling. It can be difficult to provide care at home in circumstances where the person continually falls over.

> *I started to escort my mother everywhere after her fall, especially up and down stairs, but that became time-consuming and tiring. In the end, after rearranging rooms, I finally had to move my mother downstairs.*

– A Daughter

Sadly, some carers have ordered people repeatedly to sit or have even used restraint. Caregivers may feel pushed to their limits in trying to provide care to the person with dementia who constantly falls over. However, extreme reactions and bad practices are abusive, restrictive and against the law. Caregivers must find ways of coping, and the sharing of hints and tips with other carers will be beneficial.

Fed up – caregivers can feel fed up at times, which comes about through a sense of personal fatigue, fear, frustration, lack of freedom, exasperation, arguments, and more. Support groups for carers or other ways to discuss feelings can give some relief.

> *It's not easy to argue or reason with someone who'll not remember two minutes later what the shouting match was about. As far as I'm concerned, sometimes he only behaves like that to wind me up – why else would dad keep moving furniture around the place that trips me up as I go about my chores?*

– A Daughter

Feeding – carers may have to help people with dementia to eat their meals. Some days, people might feed themselves and some days they will not – or they cannot, but they would not let a carer help them either. In certain types of dementia, food may not be recognisable on account of people's inability to recognise what is being looked at, especially if the food or drink is the same colour as the plate or glass. Caregivers have to exercise patience when they feed a person as a simple meal can take much time.

> *Some practical words of advice. It can help to say what the meal is and allow her to smell the food. Don't offer food and drink alternately – you'll find that after a while when you offer a spoon, the lips will be pouted to receive the glass or cup; then when you offer the drink, the mouth will be wide open to receive the spoon.*

– Care Home Worker

For people with difficulty in swallowing but who have not reached the stage of using liquified foods, there is a risk of choking – so carers must ensure that what is being eaten has been chewed properly, and swallowed, before attempting to give another spoonful.

> ❝*For some reason, some people with dementia can take a long time to chew their food. Or some people like to eat standing up, or to take a mouthful and walk away, or to sit elsewhere from where the carer is, or to leave their plate on the table and take food from someone else's plate, which can start a row. Left to their own devices, some people will put all their drink in the food and create an inedible soup, similarly they put the biscuits in the tea or the fruit juice in the tea where it curdles and is undrinkable.*❞
>
> **– Care Home Worker**

People might use their fingers rather than cutlery to eat their food. It is better they feed themselves by how they want to eat rather than being forced to use cutlery. An individual may have forgotten how to use cutlery or find it difficult to hold. For people who can feed themselves, a range of cutlery pieces and aids are available such as appliances to help keep food on the plate, making the plate steady on the table and on other surfaces, or cutlery that helps people with arthritic hands. Coloured plates and cups or mugs may assist in the self-feeding process as finger-food items can be easier to distinguish.

Feet – people living with dementia seem to have unusual ideas about their actions and intentions, which can hamper carers. For example, consider these possible thoughts when people are being assisted in getting dressed with footwear:

- I will offer the left foot for the right shoe and the right foot for the left shoe.
- I will keep my ankles crossed at all times whilst sitting or lying and defy any attempts to uncross them when my carer wants to put on my stockings, socks, shoes, slippers or underwear.
- I will present my heel when my carer wants me to present my toes.
- I will swipe my carers across the back of the head when they bend down to clean between my toes or to cut my toenails.
- I will stand firmly on both feet and defy my carer's attempts to make me move.
- I will shuffle in my slippers and walk at a snail's pace in the house and sprint down the road the minute the front door is open.

Hands – daughters or sons who are caregivers may hardly believe the change in their parents. Hands that used to hug and hold them safely as children will be the same hands that grab and hold on to a wrist, or item of clothing, with a tenacity and strength that is unbelievable. If the person grips strongly onto an object, their fingers may have to be prised off one by one so that carers can retrieve it. When dirt accumulates under the fingernails carers have to find a way to clean the nails or to seek assistance. Also, people may have liked their fingernails painted and kept at a shapely level.

> ❝*Grabbing is particularly unhelpful when I want to dress or undress her, remove her wet knickers, or a wet pad from underneath her, especially in bed. She either behaves like she's a log of wood and rolls all in one piece nearly off the bed or she'll clutch and grab tightly on to my hands restricting the blood supply to that area so at times I cry out in agony. A trick to distract her – known to be fairly effective some of the time – is to give her an object such as a cuddly toy to hold and occupy her attention while I attend to the job in hand.*❞
>
> **– A Daughter**

Incontinence of urine – carers have to deal with the effects of this type of incontinence in people with dementia. A washing machine and a tumble dryer or a drying area are assets to the household, along with a plentiful supply of replacement clothing and bedding. As the weather does not always allow for the drying of sheets outside, or people may live in a flat, the smell of urine can hang around for some time.

> *After a while, and despite all attempts at toilet training, there are days when I eat, sleep, drink, live and breathe urine! It pervades the atmosphere and soaks into everything it comes into contact with.*

– A Family Member

Individuals with dementia may or may not know they have urinated on themselves, or they may have an awareness, but no idea what to do next. They can become agitated or weepy on account of it, or they may sit quietly all day with a soaking wet pad. During the course of that day, the wet pad will smell more and more offensive and may begin to harbour bacteria that can lead to a urine infection.

Insomnia – a potential problem for carers and the person receiving care. In some dementias, sleeping patterns change and day can become night for that person but not for the carer.

> *I didn't believe she'd sleep for long during the day. I let her have a little nap after lunch thinking soon she'll wake up and I'll have tea ready. I'm watchful and pottering about quietly at first because she needs the sleep, but when the sleeping goes on for too long I start to make a lot of noise hoping she'll wake up. If that doesn't work, I might gently shake her while calling her name, but then I have to spend the next ten minutes explaining who I am, and how and why I'm in her house. By then it's late afternoon, I still haven't napped, and she's raring to go once she's had her tea. The night's drawing in and I wonder again if I'll get any sleep tonight.*

– A Daughter

Jealousy – is what caregivers may feel for anyone whose parents are ageing and living well.

> *I expected a mighty hand to strike me down on account of my admission of jealousy. Friends, family members and people say things like, 'You're so good to have your mother living with you.' Or, 'It must be such a joy for her.' Or, 'It's a pity more children aren't like you instead of putting their parents into a home.' These are people who've not had to look after an ageing relative with dementia or whose parents are at rest in some churchyard or urn.*

– A Daughter

> ❝*I know it's a silly thing to say, I feel I should be damned to hell for thinking it, but I sometimes feel real hatred for anyone whose parents are elderly and still live well, or whose parents do not have any chronic illness, or have even moved away to Spain or abroad, or have died.*❞
>
> – A Daughter

Joints – become very stiff quite early on, and without much warning, if they are not used or ill-used. All the joints from the neck to the large toes can seize up, becoming painful and limited in their use. Possible relief, or prevention to delay problems with joints, can come about through some form of daily activity such as walking, swimming if possible, massaging people's joints and limbs especially following a bath, or a wash, or even when sitting together, or when the caregiver puts the person to bed at night. There is a suggestion that both passive exercises such as can be done while a person is sitting and active exercises little and often – whatever can be managed – during the day may be enough to keep the joints from seizing up.

Kindness – carers need not be afraid to accept the kindness of friends, neighbours and strangers. An act of kindness done to a caregiver might be just the thing necessary to soothe the heart after a testing moment. It means a lot to be gently spoken with, to have a hug, or a reassuring touch, or a kind look.

Lifting: moving and handling – must never be attempted unless carers have been trained or can have help by someone who is trained. If carers try to manage at home, lifting can cause injury to both the caregiver and the person with dementia.

Training in the safe way to lift and carry loads, including the safe lifting of people, is demonstrated and taught in care homes and hospitals. Some dementia care organisations have begun to offer this training to their support workers.

Masking the truth – caregivers may have to be inventive or withhold the truth on a number of issues. For example, people with dementia may ask about a deceased partner or child, so carers will have to recognise when to mask the truth. Some situations are complicated and caregivers may find themselves becoming more creative especially when a query is repeated to the point where they want to scream out the truth and make the questions stop.

> ❝*I'm sorry to admit to masking of the truth. It's to do with trying to avoid making my parent more anxious and also to do with taking the easier route for me.*❞
>
> – A Daughter

> ❝*She asks every day if our Norman has had his tea, and I say, 'Yes, Mother, he's had his tea and gone out again.' The fact that our Norman has been dead for years, and if he was alive wouldn't give a toss about her anyway, is not relevant. I want to have a peaceful, contented woman instead of a distressed one.*❞
>
> – A Daughter

Nakedness – some people with dementia seem to develop the habit of removing all or bits of their clothing for no apparent reason.

> *I tried various ways of preventing disrobing from happening like putting my mother's blouses on back to front, giving her jumpers with turtle necks, putting on more than two layers of clothing. I changed the types of fabric in case it was something irritating my mother's skin; I changed the type of washing powder and conditioner for the same reason. I tried placing small cuddly objects in each of my mother's hands, which worked for a while but I forgot to replace the objects after a meal or sometimes they got lost. I tried distracting my mother by giving her things to do and occupying her hands; I tried sitting with her and reading to her, but all the while I was trying these things, mother kept taking her clothes off and fighting me when I tried to put them back on. It made no difference what the weather was like. Some days my mother would be agitated during this activity, and some days she appeared calmly determined. Many days I was in tears when people came round and found mother looking uncared for, unkempt, and like 'a mad woman', which is what I felt they thought. And one day as suddenly as it started, it stopped.*
>
> **– A Daughter**

Nourishment – especially crucial for carers at home as they need to be as fit and healthy as possible. To give care at home demands physical and mental strength, the work is hard on body and mind. Caregivers need to eat well and regularly, and to allow time for health check-ups at the GP surgery.

> *I'm a nurse and so was my mother. We believed in healthy living and eating, we took vitamins and mineral supplements as we felt the way foods were produced, many nutrients would be lost by the time we got to cooking them. I noticed when mum was getting on in age and no longer able to be as active or concerned about what she ate, she became listless, sleepy, low in mood. When she remembered to take the supplements she perked up. I continued giving them to her in the early years of her dementia.*
>
> **– A Daughter**

Pain – an important factor to consider. Due to their confusion, people with dementia may not be able to communicate hurt or pain in words to carers or to be understood in another way.

Carers must be alert to people's body language that describes pain to them, for example, by a change in posture or a preference for a specific posture; a change in the way people walk or hold themselves when walking; a grimace or a sound when certain fingers, toes or limbs are moved; a reluctance to move certain parts of the body, or to swallow, or to chew; or the eyes watering when people have swallowed a lump of food or something.

Other signs of pain to look out for include a rise in body temperature indicated by hot skin; a painful look on a person's face when using the toilet to try and urinate or defecate, which may account for a reluctance to open the bowels. Urine that smells offensive can mean an infection or dehydration. Headaches are difficult to ascertain but at times people may have been keeping their eyes closed when usually open, or keeping their head very still, which could cause the problem. Wheezing and a constant chesty cough can cause pain in the chest. Lack of movement gives rise to stiffness in the joints, or cramps that will cause pain when an attempt is made to move them. Limbs that are not walked or exercised regularly will get locked in certain positions and knees may stay bent so any attempt to straighten people up or correct their posture will be painful.

Carers need to tell a GP when they notice signs and symptoms of pain so the doctor can prescribe medication or advise on pain relief or physiotherapy. In some cases of urinary infection, which can be observed as a rapid increase in the confusional state, the doctor should be called immediately.

If carers decide to buy over-the-counter remedies, they must be aware these can have a damaging interaction with medication the person is taking – so tell the pharmacist about all prescription medicines the person takes.

Patience – carers need to cultivate key aspects of patience such as acceptance of waiting; perseverance; ability to resist provocation; calmness; endurance; choosing to ignore hindrances and anything that causes annoyance. The quality of patience is necessary when caring for people with all forms of dementia amid the realities of daily living. The constant repetition, lack of comprehension, slowness, flares up of temper and unbelievable things which people say, can make carers feel their life is on hold, waiting, caught in a necessary grind and changeless routine.

Caregivers need to stay calm even when they are being emotionally and physically hurt by a loved one. A calm attitude and keeping the temper will help carers to stop from shouting at their loved ones. Carers can also try to patiently avoid speaking for people with dementia or finishing sentences – attempt to work out what they are saying.

Quietness – is to be valued at times. It is recommended that carers build quiet time for themselves into the daily routine of caring. But also carers must let the people they care for know someone is around since they are apt to become anxious. During quiet times, if possible, use meditation and relaxation techniques.

> ❝*I used time after lunch for catching up on little jobs. I guarded this period fiercely even to the point of asking visitors not to call. Mainly, I had a rest and recharged my batteries. One day I was sitting in the chair in my mother's room doing mending, while mum dosed. I must have dosed off as well and awoke with a start to find my mother staring intently at me with a worried look on her face. When I checked my watch, I realised I'd been asleep for the best part of two hours! Mother probably thought I was dead, not having seen me sit still for so long.*❞
>
> – A Daughter

Safety – Carers have to consider safety issues in the home. If the main concern is one of falling there are aids and devices on the market that can alert carers very quickly when a person is moving about, for example, an electronic mat positioned slightly away from the bed or chair and wired to an alarm system. A simple baby alarm in the person's room to wherever the carer goes keeps track of any sounds that then alerts the listener.

Safety measures need to be assessed by merit, and discussed with a specialist who does risk assessments such as an occupational therapist, and careful steps taken to minimise the risks.

Skin – carers need to look after people's skin, which may become dry and flaky. Sadly, age brings descent and skin that does not flop, pleats. The skin of an elderly person tends to dry out and is subject to pressure sores especially in bony areas.

The poor circulation responsible for dementia, heart disease, and other related conditions can cause serious ulcers on the skin especially on the sacrum – around the sacral/pelvic area – and the heels, which can be difficult to treat or cure.

Carers need to look out for skin that has been lying in one position for too long; skin that comes into contact with urine and not washed enough; skin that gets cuts, insect bites or blisters, which are not attended to or treated quickly enough; skin that flops over the top of the upper thighs leaving an area underneath, which tends to be forgotten or overzealously dried. This hidden area is prone to sweatiness, a sore groin starts to form on both sides; breasts that now sag can suffer soreness in a similar way.

Moderate use of body lotions, barrier creams, baby oils, soap preparations in the bath or wash water, and gentle regular massage of the skin can keep the skin smooth and moisturised.

Men's private parts also need careful attention as that area is prone to irritation and dryness, and can lead to painful constriction. If a catheter is involved extra care must be taken to ensure infection does not develop.

Carers may find it difficult to attend to people's private areas. They may not pay the close attention to detail that is required for thorough skin care and cleaning routines.

Sleep – if carers are to do the job properly and safely, a good night's sleep is necessary every night or some sleep at any given chance. Carers at home and carers who are employed to look after others share the common need to fully rest and be recharged by a sound night's sleep. Sleep for people who are being looked after is also essential if carers are to enjoy days free of rattiness and tired wakefulness.

❝*When I was a baby and not sleeping through the night, my parents probably wondered if they'd ever get a good night's sleep. My nights improved as I grew older and developed, but now I'm a carer for mum I think the same thing and wonder if I'll ever sleep well. Her nights may not improve.*❞

– A Daughter

If caregivers and people with dementia experience difficulties with sleep, GPs can prescribe medication on either a short-term or long-term basis – or on a 'when required' basis. Efficient medication can ensure that everyone can sleep well. Carers may subsequently decide not to take night medication as they have to be careful if needed to perform a care service during the night.

A drawback of medication – to help with sleep or other conditions – is individuals with dementia might feel sleepy or drowsy during the day and difficult to rouse in order that carers can attend to them and provide appropriate care.

Visitors – are to be encouraged, especially family members and friends known to the individual before the dementia set in. Whether or not the person remembers other people, at least they will see a different face from the carer, and the visitor will feel good for having visited.

Visitors may encourage memories to return by their conversations and their presence. It does not matter if the visitor has to be introduced every time or if the same conversation is followed. It might be repetitive to the visitor but all may be new every time to the person with dementia.

Also, visitors may observe changes or improvements which carers might not notice as they are very close; it can help for visitors and carers to open up about changes they perceive.

> **"**If you visit regularly you become acquainted with other visitors. One of them told me my wife was always crying and agitated after I left, and staff found her difficult to manage or settle. When I asked the staff why they didn't tell me they said they thought I'd get upset too and wanted to spare me. They knew she would eventually calm down even though it took time and lots of one-to-one attention.**"**
>
> **– A Husband**

If people with dementia have had a regular faith practice and previously attended a sacred space, members of their religious group can make visits or provide a special service.

> **"**Whatever people's faith, it's useful if someone from their own religion visits. For example, if loved ones have been attending a church, the priest, or vicar, or members of the church group will want to visit. If they like hymns and prayers, someone else might come and present these aloud, and maybe 'Songs of Praise' will be on TV. They can be given taped favourite hymns for use quietly in their rooms or for use with headphones.**"**
>
> **– A Carer**

Birthdays are an important celebration and a good time to encourage visitors. Family members may say that the birthday mum or dad does not know what is going on – but they might know precisely what is happening on any given moment during that particular day.

Weight – when people with dementia become inactive or bedridden, a hoist is a good practical aid for easy handling. This aid can be used whether a person is heavy or not but it is cumbersome and will need storing where it cannot be tripped over. Not many households have the space for a hoist. Even if there is space for a hoist, carers may not have the ability to manoeuvre it as required. Carers need to maintain people's body weight at a size with which they can cope.

> "It's all well and good saying mother loves her chocolates, but when I have to lift her, if she falls or I have to perform some activities with her, then it may be too late for her to start losing weight."

– A Daughter

Yes – is a good word to know and a good answer to questions from people who are concerned and who ask caregivers if they would like help with something or further support for the person with dementia.

Yield – carers must acknowledge when they know they have had enough especially if they are caring for someone at home on their own, or having to divide time between family and work. It can take caregivers a long time and much soul-searching to get to the realisation of weariness, but there comes a time when the professionals have to be called in. Carers can talk to a GP, or their siblings, their children, or anyone who can improve the situation on their behalf. When carers are at the end of their limits, they need to take action even if it means finding a care home; any personal guilt can be dealt with later on.

> "I'm sorry to say that since my husband developed full-blown dementia, I've turned into a new woman. He was a very controlling man and became more so as he started on the road to his current state. In our marriage, I did everything to please him and carried on doing so especially when the realisation set in that he was becoming more and more dependent. When the carer used to come for two hours twice a week so I could get the shopping or have some time off, I used to feel guilty for leaving him as I knew he'd be calling for me and I'd hurry through the activities. One day my daughter-in-law encouraged me to see that I was neither helping him nor myself by being anxious and downtrodden and consumed with the effort of his care. As the dementia progressed the family helped me to decide on a care home on account of the mental and physical toll that caring for him was taking out on me. I was not living well with his dementia. It's been one year since he was placed in the care home, which I and the family visit often and get involved in any issues that arise, but I leave there with a light heart in the certainty he does not know me anymore. The care home is his family now and if the worst was to happen he'd be among people and friends with whom he has come to be more familiar. I've joined a couple of dementia charities, taken up bowling, and spend a lot more time with the grandchildren than I did before when their granddad was taking up so much of my time. I'm ageing gracefully now and enjoying it instead of the despairing and depressive future that I had envisaged for myself with my beloved but dementing husband."

– A Wife

Golden Rules

BEFORE DOING ANYTHING, carers can let people with dementia know what they intend to do.

CARERS NEED to let the person with dementia give some help as much as they are able, and to give praise and encouragement even for the slightest bit of assistance they have been given.

PEOPLE WITH DEMENTIA will lose interest in giving assistance so any help they could have given to a carer will be lost. Carers must try not to rush through tasks, yet also not take too long.

CARERS MUST make things easy for themselves, especially after a hard day. For example, if a person with dementia is tired and wants to go to bed in their day clothes or if they want to stay in bed or in their pyjamas all day, let it be.

DO NOT OVERFEED people with dementia. It is possible to live well without overfeeding. The lack of mobility and exercise will put weight on their lower joints and could make walking difficult.

WHEN THINGS ARE PROGRESSING WELL and caregivers have the necessary help and support if they need it, they usually feel they have made the right decision to care for an individual at home. But suffering from dementia does not exclude the possibility of a physical mishap or the person needing to go into hospital. Do not self-blame.

CARERS MUST have a way of letting someone know they are solely responsible in providing care for another person. That information is useful if the carer has an accident or will be unable to care for the person at the expected time.

CARERS MUST listen to their own body and mind, and be attentive to their own well-being. Carers must acknowledge when they have had enough.

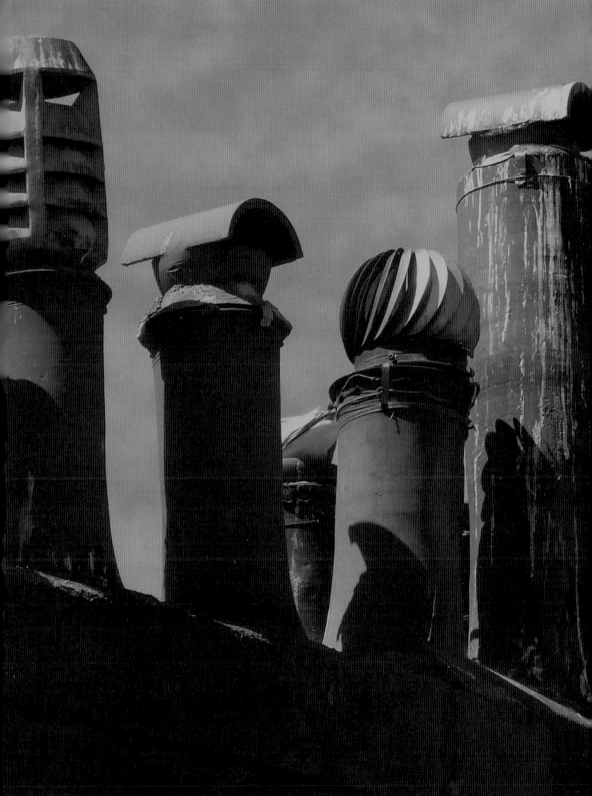

In hospitals, caring for the physical and mental needs of a person with dementia may require more space than is available for the safe working layout of the ordinary ward. There is so much equipment already in the ward; it could be problematic and expensive to add hoists, stand aids, wheelchairs, rollators, manual handling equipment that people may need plus individual items such as Zimmer frames, walking frames, commodes.

As with other patients, those with dementia have the basic right to be nourished and have personal care given to them at their most vulnerable such as when they are away from familiar surroundings and possibly undergoing physical or medical treatment of which they are unable to make sense.

Carers state that there needs to be careful thought by staff in relation to visiting times and the positioning of people with dementia in the ward with regard for their safety and particular needs.

Visiting hours suggested by some hospitals allow staff the time in which to attend to their duties without interference from visitors and family – but that resource of visitors could be beneficial to an understaffed ward and ensure the needs of people with dementia are met.

A-Z and reflections for carers

❝My aunt caught an infection from the day centre she attended twice a week and had to be hospitalised on account of a breathing problem. During her stay at the hospital she developed pneumonia, which extended the stay and caused more disorientation. We visited every day so she could see a face she knew but we were always apprehensive before the visit in case something else had come up that would set her back. Some of the staff took time to explain the menu list to see what she wanted, or we would choose for her when we were there, but she never was a big eater and ate even less in the hospital. We spoke to the ward sister about the good versus negative effects of putting her in a side room. In the end she was placed in a side room with the door ajar so she could hear what was going on around her, and as there was no chance of her getting up and walking about it seemed the better option. In her room we could feed her and chat to her more loudly than we could when she was in the six-bedder ward, and we'd keep her entertained without spoiling the visit for someone else. She returned home with a sore on her bottom and needed the district nurses over until it healed up, which took its time because of the pads and the urine.❞

– A Niece

❝My mum fell over a chair in her own house and broke her hip; she did not suffer from dementia at the time but when she was discharged from hospital, her stay there seemed to have started a process of mental deterioration.❞

– A Daughter

Information – if people with dementia have to be admitted to hospital it is best for caregivers to remain until they are sure the staff have all the relevant information concerning patients. Carers must clearly communicate with staff as, after they have gone home, the person left behind in hospital may not be able to answer questions. The change from their familiar environment can confuse people, they could be worse for weeks afterwards.

Even with the best intentions of staff, the level of dependency that a dementia patient displays might not always be catered for in a busy surgical or medical ward. Understandably, nurses and doctors will want the patient with dementia to receive the best possible care. A reality may be that wards are not adequately equipped for the additional work required, so there is a double challenge to provide appropriate, effective and individual care.

> ❝Someone came in the other day and told us off because she found two cups and a glass with drinks by her nan's bed and thought we'd not persevered with her when she said she didn't want a drink. We do try to find out what the patient prefers and make sure they get it. But we can't assume that what is liked one day will be accepted the next time it's offered. When we offer what people like and has been prepared for them, they may say no or refuse to drink it but minutes later proceed to drink the lot. Some days they'll let us feed them and other days they'll push our hands away and refuse to eat or drink. We've found that if people are not crowded too much and we offer little and often, they'll eventually drink the whole amount. But it all takes time and hot drinks and food get cold.❞
>
> **– A Nurse**

If carers at home are elderly and suffering from their own physical complaints, it can be a struggle to go to the hospital every day to make sure loved ones are receiving the right care. It can be difficult to find out who is the correct staff member to ask about the progress of a partner with dementia. There may also be a deference shown to authority figures such as doctors, especially among people of the older generation, which prevents them from asking too many questions in order to reassure themselves that doctor knows best.

Hospital staff may well be glad that carers come to visit their patient and might leave the feeding to them – although that can mean carers will worry about what happens when they leave or cannot visit.

An ideal situation, suggested by carers, would be a ward like a care home ward that looks after dementia patients coping with a physical illness. Ideally the staff working there will have been specially trained. The hospital can be a confusing place for people with dementia and if they find themselves in the Accident and Emergency department (A&E) there may be multiple complications.

> ❝A person with dementia who is brought into a busy A&E department can cause disruption. A&E – with its many cubicles, doctors and nurses rushing about, ambulance staff arriving and delivering more and more people, emergency admissions placing anyone waiting lower and lower down the list for attention – might be the most confusing and bewildering place for someone with dementia. The injured and their relatives are stressed out, children are crying or screaming, then into that chaos comes a person with dementia, confused and needing physical treatment.

It would be ideal if there was someone who could provide one-to-one care until they are seen, or a room where they could be accommodated away from the busyness – but that's in a perfect world and we're not there yet. The care for people with dementia becomes critical and demanding because of the disruption they are causing. They have tried to get off the trolley, they won't or can't answer when asked their name, they're unable to give details about pain or where they may be hurting, they're weeping, calling for a son or daughter, and becoming singly or doubly incontinent and refusing to be taken to the toilet or to be led away. Frustration runs high as other patients in distress are looking to us to calm people down or asking us to do something with them. In the absence of information a decision has to be taken about appropriate action and subsequent placement. If relatives or someone who knows the dementia patient cannot be found, the patient has to be housed in any ward where there is a vacancy until such time as a relative turns up. If it's discovered they live on their own, there's no way they can be returned until we have a case assessment meeting to discuss and decide future action.

Even if they live in a care home, it may not be practicable to return them there if the aftercare required is beyond the scope of the home's competence. So a different place will have to be sought. The patient will have to remain in the hospital until a suitable home is found. The choice of ward depends on the injury sustained in the initial stages, but when they have recovered and are over the worst and need convalescence, they may have to be removed from the ward where they have become familiar and placed in another unfamiliar setting – the confusion can start all over again. The longer it takes to find a suitable placement puts a strain on the bed situation and they become known by the unfavourable term as a bed blocker. **"**

– Nurse on an A&E Department

Quirks – if a person with dementia is going to stay in hospital, it is worthwhile passing on to staff information about any habits or peculiarities they might have. The carer can mention features of a person's character that could make life more comfortable for the patient as well as the staff. This information helps people to have a more enjoyable stay in hospital.

"*I gave hospital staff information about her morning, evening and night-time routines, the fact that she only hears when she has her glasses on, and she prefers her pudding before the main meal. I mentioned there are some foods she eats better without her dentures. She gets up to answer the doorbell every time the phone rings. When she walks around in circles it means she wants to use the toilet. She's partially sighted and able to feed herself but she still needs a push start at the beginning of the meal.* **"**

– A Daughter

Carers should write down all their observations as accurately as they can recall them such as whether a person chokes on any food that is not cut up really small, or is better off with mashed foods, and any other unusual characteristics they may have noticed creeping in to a person's personality along with the dementia. Carers know their loved ones better than anyone, and hospital staff find these reports helpful. It could enhance the care a patient receives when carers are away.

Information that is valuable to hospital staff includes facts such as whether the person wears a hearing aid, false teeth, wears glasses or is usually mute, has a poor appetite and needs feeding, or needs help to use the toilet.

When a planned admission has been booked, a pre-admission medical assessment is invited before any medical or surgical procedure takes place. This assessment is done in order to ascertain the level of physical debility, mental aptitude and what care is already in place, if anything, for the patient and the person looking after them at home.

The pre-admission may also be the beginning of a discharge plan, and potential problems on discharge can be flagged up. Problems on discharge include whether or not the carer looking after the patient will be able to meet their personal and physical needs and, more practically, to meet needs such as cooking for them, managing them on a daily basis, and knowing where to get help.

If the admission is for day surgery then there may not be a pressing need for such a detailed report, but for a longer stay then more personal details are useful to decide on issues such as whether patients would be better off in a side room or feel less isolated in the main ward.

Golden Rules

CARERS NEED to write down anything they think hospital staff should know that may be relevant. It can make a difference to the patient as to how the stay is endured or enjoyed.

CARERS should write down the name of the ward, the doctor or specialist and, if possible, key staff who will be in charge of the person admitted to their care.

CARERS CAN ASK if they may be able to assist with feeding when they visit. It may also be possible to have their own snack at the same time.

CARERS SHOULD take time to thank hospital staff for all their work and kindness towards their loved ones.

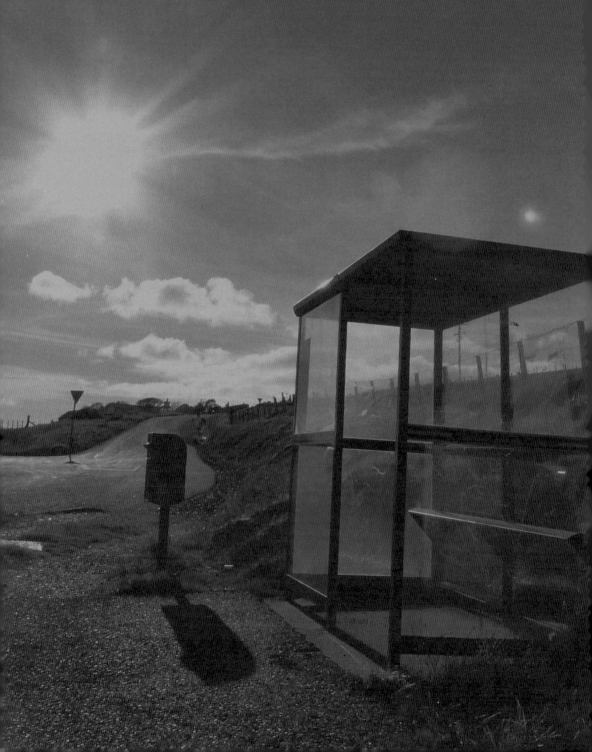

CHAPTER 13 — CHOOSING A CARE HOME; THE CARE HOME

Admission to a care home may not happen overnight. Prior to the placement of people with dementia in a care home, their primary caregivers will have had hard decisions to make. The day may come when the main caregiver has had enough, cannot cope, and a choice has to be taken around care. Everyone in the immediate circle of family or friends should be informed this decision comes from a sense of the carer not being able to manage any longer – and something must be done. Sometimes, no one will have recognised caregivers are being pushed to their limits – and extreme actions might result.

> " *I cringe with shame every time I think about what I did to my mother. I finally decided to place her in a home we had both been looking at and which seemed to be the best of the lot. On the day we were leaving to go, I got her to help me, at least to be in the same room with me while the packing was taking place. All the while I kept talking to her saying how she'd soon settle in and about the friends she'd make in the home. I was hoping the loss of memory and the confusion over times and places would serve her in good stead and she'd not remember what the trip really entailed. After arriving at the home, the staff let us unpack and settle her in her new room. While mum was enjoying a cup of tea I went off to speak to the manager and complete a few forms and fill in some more details that had come to mind since the last time we were there. When it came time to leave, mum came to the door with me saying goodbye to the staff and was trying to follow me out the door. So I said, 'You wait here, mum, I'm just going to the car to get those sweets you like.' And I ran away. Weeks later, and I still had not returned. Although I phone quite often, I've not gone back yet because if I visit her I'll only have to leave her again. It's dreadful I know, but I can't seem to face it.* "

– A Daughter

> " *My sister took my mother round to me, said she was popping out to the shops, and went on holiday abroad. That may sound a bit unreasonable – but I think she felt no one listened to her or we thought she was whingeing.* "

– A Daughter

Every member of a family can help in choosing a care home for their loved one, listening well and taking everyone's views into account. When one family member makes the selection, there could be recriminations if a parent with dementia is felt to be wrongly placed. Alternatively, one person could ask someone who is not emotionally involved for help in assessing the standards and practices of a care home.

> " *It was no easy task to choose a home from the variety in the area for my mum. Visiting many and different care homes to find the right one was emotionally draining because the standards can be diverse. Also, you may feel intimidated when asking a lot of questions and can be made to feel that you have unreasonable expectations.* "

– A Daughter

> ❝My sons made it clear they wanted no part of my decision to send their stepfather to a care home and wouldn't be helping me to choose one. Their relationship with him was cool. In the early days of our marriage they'd lived with their father and only heard about their stepfather's treatment of me when I chose to tell them. In the latter stages when physical illness married up with the Alzheimer's, and contributed to his bad temper, his treatment of me got worse and I could no longer put up with it. They literally said, 'You made your bed…' They advised me to leave him. I had to take a friend with me to investigate the homes suggested by the social worker, when he was ill in hospital, and having him back home was out of the question.❞
>
> – A Wife

To ensure the right care home is chosen, carers must be clear about all the facts concerning the person with dementia and also consider other factors such as visiting. Carers can read up about selected care homes on the Care Quality Commission (CQC) website.

Depending on the physical and mental needs of the person with dementia, it may be necessary to re-evaluate suggestions about care provision, and a care home with nursing may be a better option than a residential care home.

A care home with nursing may house residents some of whom experience difficulty in managing activities of daily living. Nursing homes have registered nurses on their staff.

A residential home may house residents who are not yet dependent on staff for their needs – meaning people can feed themselves, know when they need to use the toilet, find their way around and perform self-care with little help. Some residents may be able to go out on their own.

A care home may serve a dual purpose and house residents with mixed abilities. Care homes may accept a couple and accommodate them in a double room so they can attempt to carry on as if they were at home.

> ❝This double room seems to work well and mum can carry on nagging dad as she's always done! He in turn can be seen doing little things for her, and they can hold hands together on the settee.❞
>
> – A Son and Daughter

When choosing a care home, consider all-round comfort. If individuals are housed in a care home that maintains good standards and provision throughout their journey into full-blown dementia, they may be able to stay on.

At a care home, the manager and a member of staff will meet with the main caregiver to record aspects of the life and care needs of the person with dementia. It is important that relatives and loved ones provide background information so staff can begin to work more knowingly with the resident.

Primary carers and family members need to talk about location of a care home, walking or driving distances and the availability of transport. Care homes with remote access may pose difficulties if the visiting carers are elderly themselves and have to depend on public transport. Mobile phones have made it possible for close contact between the carer and the care home.

> **❝***Distance might lend enchantment to the view, but it can be a case of out of sight out of mind! Both statements need to be carefully considered when choosing a home for your relative.*❞
>
> **– Care Home Staff**

There are key questions carers can consider when thinking about the location of a care home:

- Will I be physically able to travel to the care home if it is at a distance from where I live?
- Who else other than me will visit the home and how often?
- What transport is available?
- Who will take me to the care home on my loved one's birthday or special anniversaries?
- Will I be able to visit often enough to keep up to date on care provision at the home?
- Will distance stop me from providing help with feeding, or sharing the company of my loved one?

> **❝***Frequent visits show support both for the staff and your loved one. I think about those relatives who allowed distance to be the reason they didn't become involved and then raised a hue and cry when something happened. Family members might start to move away from home when dementia threatens the parent. Some have been known to leave the country.*❞
>
> **– Care Home Staff**

Golden Rules

WHEN THE PRIMARY CARER visits a care home or residential home to assess suitability, it is useful to reserve judgement for a few days in order to fully examine personal emotions, feelings and realities surrounding the final choice.

BEFORE CHOOSING A CARE HOME, it is advisable to visit potential places more than once and at different times. Never judge the care a home can give on the first visit; take time to understand how the care home provides its service, how many people it houses.

AT THE INITIAL VISIT, never condemn a care home on any smell emanating from it. People may think the elderly always smell of urine and so will the care home. Though the smell in a care home may be an indicator of the standard and level of care to be expected, it could be the home has been caught on a day when staff have had to care for more residents with incontinence than usual. The home may also encourage pets, especially rabbits, which can leave a lingering after-smell.

NEVER JUDGE a care home on the grounds of inactivity. Residents who are sitting in armchairs may just be tired after an exercise session or after lunch when a sleep is very welcome.

PREPARE QUESTIONS in advance of visiting a care home and try to get these answered by the person in charge. The carer, family members and friends can be shown round and may even see the room that will house the person with dementia. Primary carers know the person best and will be aware if they would prefer a room with a view of the street or the garden.

UNDERSTAND the reason for chairs arranged in a circle in the communal area – enabling residents to see each other, or to participate in a group activity, or to watch the television.

TRY TO UNDERSTAND the reason for some residents walking about looking unkempt. A reason may be that staff are facilitating freedom of movement, or they are refraining from struggling with a resident who has refused to allow a change of clothing.

TRY TO APPRECIATE why staff may follow residents around and feed them in the corridor, or standing up. Staff may only be trying to ensure a resident who is unwilling to comply with dining room etiquette does manage to drink and eat well.

HELP STAFF ease the transition into a care home by letting them know of people's personal traits or quirks, likes and dislikes, and lifestyle.

ALL CARE HOMES would have been inspected by the Care Quality Commission and its reports are available online. If you do not own a computer, ask a friend or ask at the local library for help to use the internet.

The care home

A-Z and reflections for carers

Agencies – specialise in providing excellent, trained carers. All care staff must be screened for suitability by the Disclosure and Barring Service (DBS), which alerts potential employers to people on a register who have a record of an offence that makes them unsuitable for the job of caring. Agency staff may be used by care homes in an emergency or when there is a shortage of their own staff.

Care staff – get paid to work in an environment where care is required on a 24-hour basis for those who are unable to care for themselves. Staff who have worked for years in care homes may tell visitors they love their job. In the care setting a bond can be formed. Staff are likely to take the time to show affection and friendship, they help residents to lead fulfilling days spanning the stages of dementia and dependency, and they value residents in their care.

The common goal of care staff will be to do the best they can for the person in their charge or for whom they have a responsibility.

By staff making time to listen to and involve relatives and friends in people's care, and by working in partnership, it is possible to develop a loving and caring community, beneficial to all.

Care homes may employ care staff who have National Vocational Qualifications (NVQ) in Health and Social Care which prove they have studied and developed their skills under supervision and have good practical experience. What care homes must have in place as a matter of legality is ongoing training for all staff.

Staff in care homes are responsible to ensure all residents receive equality of care provision. People with dementia in care homes must receive quality care and best practice. Full-blown dementia care is demanding work and staff may be unable to become as deeply involved with their clients as relatives would wish as the focus is on care.

Residents each have different habits and needs. Care staff can learn the individual needs of every person they look after and consider each person in their own right. Some family members might feel their loved ones warrant added attention or give specific instructions but staff must always consider moral and legal requirements.

> "It can be difficult to cater for the different needs of so many individuals on any given day and to also cater for the socialising that is important to them all. Someone's mum might want to stay in bed all day, despite having been cajoled by the staff to get up for lunch or even afternoon tea – but she does not. So what more can we do? If someone's dad refuses to get undressed and prefers to walk around all day in his pyjamas, what more could we do? The powers of staff to go beyond what is reasonable coercion are limited. We have no magic powers. The care home becomes their home. If a family member such as a daughter or son couldn't make their parent do anything they didn't want to do at home, what more can they expect from us the staff? People might say that they give us permission to force or bully their mum into doing something, but we'd tell them we won't do it. We have a relationship to maintain with the person that could be marred if we came on heavy-handed, despite their permission. And they'd be the first ones to complain if an incident occurred because we were doing what they asked us to do."

– **Care Home Staff**

> "On one visit to the home my mum was living in, I thought she was being neglected because when I went she was still in bed when the others were having lunch, and it seemed she'd been left alone. When I asked her why she was still in bed she couldn't give me an answer. I felt at the time my mum was not being cared for properly and wondered if we should take her away. Did we have problems with the home before? Not really, and we were previously satisfied my mum was treated as an individual and not part of a mass population. It turned out she'd had a restless night and was allowed to lie-in thereby making everything later than normal."

– **A Son**

Core Training – carers and staff who work in care homes registered by the Care Quality Commission must receive regular training and keep that training updated. Staff undergo training in subjects such as infection control, first aid, food safety, health and safety, moving and handling, fire safety, vulnerable adult awareness – also known as safeguarding. All staff are expected to practise what is being taught, and to be aware of the legal consequences of their actions if they do not deliver quality care and safe care. A care home may encourage its staff to take an added interest in subjects that fall under the domain of trained staff, for example, medication administration.

Duties – staff may also provide indirect care and they can be engaged in roles such as in the laundry, in the kitchen, in the office, in the garden. Everyone in the care home contributes to care.

> "When I first placed my mum in the nursing home, me and my husband did a real big shop and bought easy-fit day clothes, nighties, bed jackets, socks, slippers, toiletries. The manager asked us to make sure mum's name was on the items, which we did, and every time after that we made sure everything was labelled. That seems to be the best way to ensure nothing gets lost or misplaced or worn by other residents."

– **A Daughter**

Entertainment – care homes may allow local schools to send one or two of their sixth-formers to assist staff with activities. Residents might enjoy listening to tapes of comedy greats of the 50s and 60s, or to the work of other entertainers. The television is popular for talent shows and game shows, and residents can become so engrossed in these shows they will laugh at the jokes or shout out an answer to questions.

Other entertainment is provided by photographs such as putting up a picture board with residents' pictures taken at special events. Carers may try to remember people's birthdays and send cards, bake cakes, give presents and make a fuss so everyone in the home has the chance to join in the celebration.

> *One resident loved dressing up and dancing; this resident sang every carol with the kids from the local school when they came round at Christmas.*

– Care Home Staff

> *Visitors may bring in their pets or there may be special sessions with pets that residents really love.*

– Care Home Worker

Exercise – to stimulate mind and body. In some care homes an activity coordinator is employed, or the staff might organise activities. Typical exercises might include gentle stretching; movement to music; gardening; yoga; board games; reminiscence. Other services might include head and hand massage, or body massage if allowed. Some care homes employ people to treat residents' hands and nails as part of a therapy session.

> *There are activities available. But some days residents can be tired, not in the mood, or uninterested; or staffing is short. That could be the very day we get an unannounced visit from the CQC or a relative turns up and asks why is there no activity going on for residents.*

– Care Home Staff

Meals for staff – carers in care homes may be allowed to purchase their lunch, or there might be a facility that allows staff to use a fridge or a microwave. Care homes might allow staff to sit with residents and have a snack with them if that will encourage a poor eater. Staff might be forbidden to eat food prepared for the residents – even if it means food is going to be thrown away – and if this rule is disobeyed it could form part of a disciplinary procedure.

No – a popular word that may be used by people with dementia. Do not always believe people if they say they have not eaten that day or had nothing to drink, or not been out for a walk with carers. The truth is probably different as they would be given regular meals and drink. Also, time-permitting they may go out for walks with the staff. If relatives are concerned and want to check out the story, they can ask another resident or a regular visitor for their impression.

> ❝ *YES is also the opposite of NO and seemingly turns mother into a liar that could get me into trouble. When I visit and inquire if she enjoyed the squash that I've seen on the bedside locker, she says, 'Yes.' I'll ask if she'll eat the cottage pie I've seen on the menu for dinner; she says, 'Yes.' Before I leave I'll ask whether she's been to the toilet today; she says, 'Yes.' But I worry I could see her in an undercover programme on TV and find she's actually a victim of neglect, dehydrated, and suffering from malnutrition, and I hadn't noticed.* ❞

– A Daughter

Questions and realities – care staff may not always have the time or the energy to be as clear as possible about questions and queries that visitors might pose. For example, if carers on shift are asked about clothing from some time ago belonging to a relative, they may not know anything about it. The carer that day might be from an agency or a new member of staff. Staff may need to make further inquiries before they can respond to questions. The care home should be able to give an explanation after specific queries but it helps to have patience, allowing time for the home to look into the matter and report back.

Regular care – a one-to-one experience of care is probably the relationship that works best for a person with dementia where their needs – emotional, physical and psychological – will be catered for individually by regular carers on a daily basis.

Relief staff – care homes may keep a list of staff known as bank staff or relief workers who can be called at fairly short notice.

Shifts – can be from six hours up to fourteen hours day or night. When there is a staff shortage, care staff may work many days one after the other, but this can result in tiredness and poor concentration.

Specialist staff – such as general or mental health nurses must undergo refresher courses in safe medication administration, dressing techniques, management and legal issues, mental capacity assessment, and in other subjects and practices relevant to their job. If staff are not qualified to do a procedure, they will know another qualified staff member whom they can call in, or they can refer on the resident with dementia to a service outside of the home.

All staff working in care homes should provide evidence of their qualifications and proof of their registration in the NHS. Staff must be familiar with training requirements and their responsibilities plus demonstrate their knowledge and experience of caring for people with dementia.

> ❝ *I was always interested in looking after people and used to go after school to help out at the local nursing home with feeding and chatting. So I felt when I left school I could work as a carer. I got the job mainly based on my past experiences and involvement with the elderly. I didn't realise training would be so intense, and the work so hard. As part of the Induction I was allowed to shadow staff who were experienced. They made it look easy, I thought I could do it when left on my own. As a trial, they said to me to get one resident up, washed, dressed and ready for breakfast. (The ethos of the house meant we were to involve residents in choosing their own clothes and basically go at their own pace.) It took me two hours! She wouldn't answer when I showed her the clothes, then she refused to dress herself in the choices we made. She refused to do anything for herself and I ended up doing it all for her. She had to have late breakfast in her room, and staff said she played me up because I was new!* ❞

– Young Carer in a Care Home

Wages – for care staff are often low, and may not include extra pay for weekends or bank holidays, known as unsocial hours.

Workplace – the work environment for care staff varies greatly. Staff's break times may be strictly adhered to, but sometimes breaks can be interrupted by a call bell. Staff will need to attend to the call bell or assist another member of staff – so they might end up losing their break period.

Workplace experiences – sharing experiences between those involved in caring for people with dementia and family members can bring greater awareness of the everyday work of staff in care homes, and of people's feelings around putting their loved ones into homes.

> *Today is just another visiting day in the care home for families and friends. I've come to see my husband who has now become a leftover of his former self. Our family couldn't be more caring. He's dressed as the man, husband, father, grandpa, brother and friend who is familiar to everyone. I'm in my senior years and turn up with my sons or the grandchildren, with yet another set of clean clothes and new slippers; the latter seem to get lost or mislaid quite regularly. Keeping my husband looking clean and smartly dressed is my way of helping him to maintain his dignity. I greet him with a kiss and steer him towards table and chairs in the dining room of the home. He's pleased to see me as he smiles warmly back at me and pulls out a chair for me being the gentleman I know him to be. He sits for a while and enjoys the homemade cake and yoghurt I've brought him but, for him, it's time to get back to work. He gets up and begins to pull tables together, aligning each one so they fit at right angles. The tables have to be dragged into position. He gets down on his knees and examines the fit but is not happy, he has to adjust and readjust one of the tables and move it this way and that way. He pushes and pulls and mumbles to himself in extreme concentration on the task. He feels behind his ear for the pencil that isn't there, and now begins to show signs of frustration and becomes agitated. He's not quite happy with the alignment but has given up on it for now and decides to wander off down the corridor.*
>
> *I've not intervened or interrupted him as I know it's best to let him carry out the procedure until he loses interest. He sets off down the corridor without a backward glance at me; on the way he pauses and wets himself.*
>
> *My husband's life with dementia now is what it is, living out his remaining years in a mixture of the past and the here and now but seemingly unconcerned about the ethics and values within which he had lived. Heartbreaking for me and all who knew him before he became ill; yet some of the man he was is still visible some days. We love him and cherish what he was and what he has become.*

– **A Wife**

> *If you were a fly on the wall, you might see it could be your mum who'll be reaching for other residents' belongings, or walking around the room touching everything, holding hands with her friend whose name she may or may not know, or on the other hand people may be oblivious to everything that is going on around them. Based on experience of residents with dementia in care homes, we understand the nature of the illness, and know how best to deal with these situations.*

– **Care Home Staff**

Golden Rules

IF PEOPLE CHOOSE to put a person with dementia under the care of someone else, think about the staff and the good work they do.

PEOPLE ARE ENTITLED to make a complaint about a carer or a care home, but this should be a valid grievance. For example, an item of jewellery might be misplaced rather than stolen by a carer; a careful investigation could avoid putting blame on staff.

BRING TO THE ATTENTION OF STAFF any perceived problems with nutrition. For example, if it is felt that a loved one is not eating or drinking well, or not being fed, then staff should be advised.

TRY TO AVOID showing love and affection through feeding cakes and chocolates to residents during visiting hours. Additional food can lead to vomiting or abdominal discomfort later on at proper mealtimes in the care home, just when staff are at their busiest. Also, in the opinion of staff, it would be preferable to maintain the person at a healthily-stable weight so people can be handled manually without the use of a hoist.

TRY NOT TO COME TO CONCLUSIONS about the behaviour of a loved one. For example, people may seem to want a snooze or a read and be quite placid in the daytime, yet they may be the very ones who keep everyone else up during the night.

SOME PEOPLE SEEM TO GET BETTER in care homes, perhaps due to shared care, the removal of stress that may occur within a one-to-one situation at home, the provision of more companionship, the possibility for proactive intervention; the creativity that brings about fun activities; the routine with the flexibility that respects the individual.

CHAPTER 14 — END STAGE

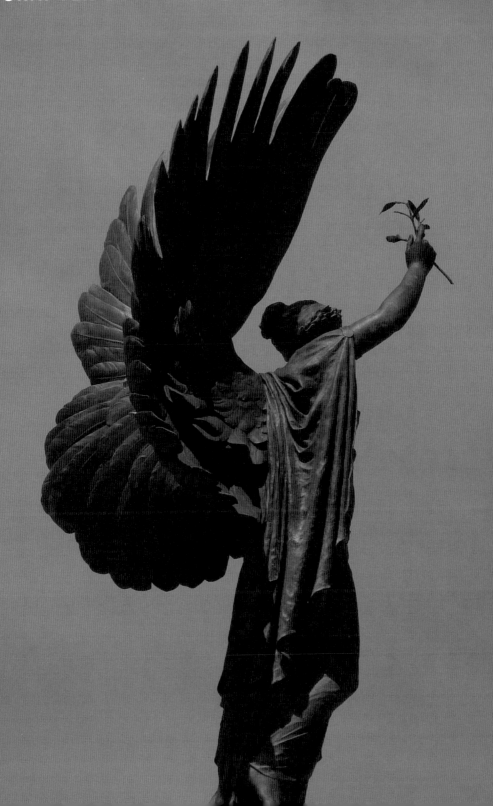

Carers might wonder how many years lie ahead for people with dementia, they may worry about the continuity of care if the caregiver dies first. There may be concerns about the quality of care and financial implications.

A-Z and reflections for carers

Death – the way dementia progresses, the way the brain eventually fails, makes it a terminal illness. Also, some carers die before the person they look after – perhaps on account of the emotional, physical and psychological toll that caring takes on them. Emotional issues especially with couples who have been married for decades create a bond they lovingly feel they cannot break. The main carer may be as old as the person who needed and received care and who died. People with dementia may never know their partner or the loved one who has been looking after them has died.

Family – sometimes family members may be at the bedside when their loved one passes away. Care home staff will inform the family so they can be with their relative around the time of death. Or sometimes family members may feel there was something more the primary carer could have done. Such judgement can cause hurt and upset to the main caregiver.

> ❝When mum died we had mixed feelings. We felt that she had died years ago when the dementia took over fully and she didn't seem to know us or know about anything. We felt sad that her life had to end like this but glad that her suffering was over. After all, your mum's your mum isn't she...❞
>
> **– A Daughter**

Funerals – sadly, sometimes the ones left behind may be in a care home themselves, they may be too frail or elderly to cope with the practicalities involved in making funeral arrangements, or to attend the funeral.

Carers and family members and friends can work together to ensure the wishes of the deceased are carried out. The views of the main caregivers deserve first consideration when arrangements are being made. Elderly carers may ask others to help with funeral arrangements. In the absence of any relatives, some care homes will take on the responsibility of dealing with practicalities surrounding a funeral.

Golden Rules

DO NOT keep inside fears of mortality – talk about worries and anxieties about end of life care with friends, partners, care home staff, GPs, faith support leaders.

CARERS OF PEOPLE WITH DEMENTIA may be able to cherish even more the time they have left together. Carers need to be aware of the impact on personal health issues if a loved one is approaching death.

TRY TO ACCEPT death. There are bereavement support services in the community that can offer counselling or other help if necessary.

IF THERE ARE ANY CONFLICTS or tensions among family members, try to resolve issues before the death of a relative. Try to make peace and help each other especially towards the end of a person's life.

CARERS SHOULD let care homes know of any difficulties that may be arising in organising funeral arrangements, or seek advice from others on how to make arrangements.

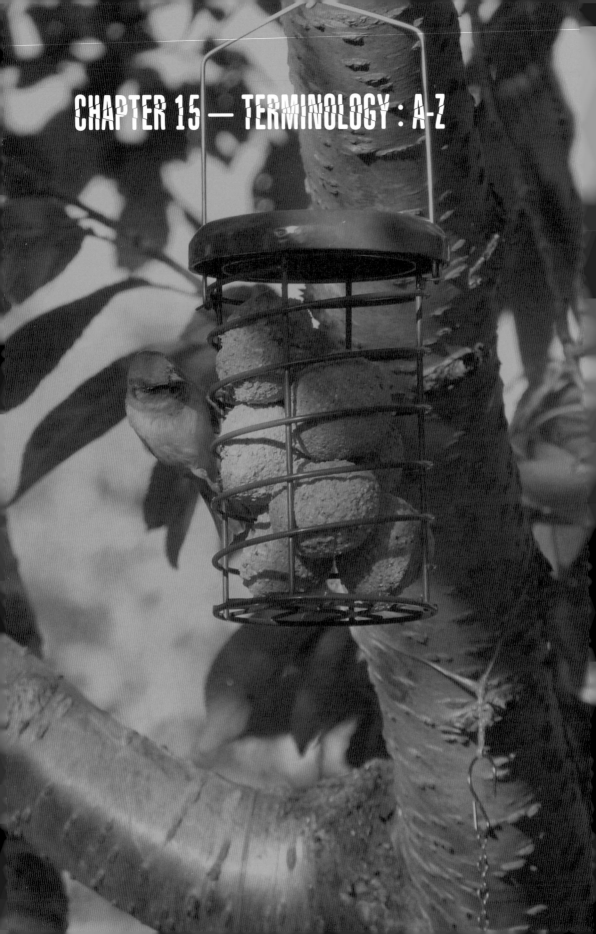

ABUSE – there is extensive legislation surrounding prevention, disclosures, training, and mechanisms at multi-discipline levels to prevent and stop abuse in all its forms wherever it may happen. Everyone in the care industry is responsible and accountable, and the law comes down heavily on perpetrators of abuse. While professional carers and support workers will receive training in caring for the vulnerable, family carers may not have access to the same service. Abuse can involve emotional, financial, sexual, physical, institutional, discriminatory factors, and may stem from ignorance, fear, misunderstanding, tiredness. Abuse may happen to the person being cared for – and to the carer.

People who are caring for a person with dementia at home can be subject to many forms of mental and physical abuse, which is sometimes kept very quiet as carers may be fearful or embarrassed. The toll that mental abuse and physical stress take on the main carer looking after relatives with dementia might result in the untimely death of that carer.

ADVOCATE – can be appointed to represent the wishes of a person with dementia if they have no one or no family to speak for them. People may be unable to state their wishes, for example, if they do not have the mental capacity, or are unable to speak up in their own right to have their requests made known and be respected. An advocate may be a friend of the person with dementia or anyone without bias who will champion a person's cause. Family members who have relinquished the task of caring may feel caught between supporting care staff, on a difficult request, and their relative.

CAPACITY – the ability to make decisions about a specific matter, at a specific time; to understand the implications of these decisions, and can communicate this to someone else. People with dementia have a fluctuating capacity and may be able to make a decison about one thing but not another such as about food choices, or about going out. Capacity specific to each issue can be considered separately.

COGNITIVE FUNCTION – different parts of the brain continually carry out simple and complex tasks giving us mental and physical skills to help us undertake the activities of daily living. In dementia these skills begin to be reduced and are ultimately lost.

CQC – Care Quality Commission, which is an independent body set up to check all health and social care services registered with them conform to and follow safe guidelines and standards. Members of the commission can visit premises as and when they like, with or without informing the establishment or service. They can interview staff, patients, relatives, or concerned people and anyone who may have made a complaint against a health service. If people have concerns about a care establishment, they can contact the CQC directly.

DBS – Disclosure and Barring Service. A recruitment safeguard via a police check on people to ensure they are not on a register that prevents them from working with vulnerable people.

DNAR/DNACPR – Do Not Attempt Resuscitation/Do Not Attempt Cardio Pulmonary Resuscitation. A DNAR form can be issued and signed by a doctor, and agreed by the person to whom it refers whilst still mentally capable to make this decision. All interested parties especially relatives should be aware of this document. It is advisable to leave this document in a visible place where it can be seen easily and quickly by a member of the emergency services. The form can be taken with the person if they have to go to hospital for any reason.

HALLUCINATIONS – hearing and seeing things that are not there.

HOLISTIC – a word used by professionals meaning carers could take into consideration the physical, mental, spiritual and recreational needs of their loved ones and try to combine these in the lifestyle of the care being provided. A holistic lifestyle may be difficult to achieve if a carer is looking after a person with dementia at home. The holistic approach to care can be expensive and take up much time, especially if it involves trips and gadgets, but it can be done and may preserve a quality of life worth striving for.

IMCA – Independent Mental Capacity Advocate. Appointed to represent people to ensure their best interests are considered when they lack the power or capacity to speak for themselves on important specific decisions. Many care homes recognise the importance of advocacy services.

LBD – Lewy body dementia. A progressive degenerative disease closely associated with Parkinson's disease. For more information, see: *www.alzheimers.org.uk* or Lewy Body Dementia Association.

LIVING WILL – advance directive, decision and statements about people's wishes especially regarding end of life care, which should always be written down. A person during the journey of dementia may be able to make changes or have changes made to a Living Will as their capacity allows.

It is advisable to take professional advice on anything that may have legal consequences. It eases the decision-making process and may even prevent family members from intervening, or ending up in court. For more information, see: *www.ageuk.org.uk*

LPA – Lasting Power of Attorney. The two types of LPA are health and welfare and property and financial affairs; a single type or both types can be made. While a person has mental capacity, they can appoint someone to protect their best interests in health and welfare matters. This power is mainly used once the person is no longer able to make these decisions for themselves. A financial LPA gives the appointee power to make decisions with financial matters. This power can also be used at the onset of some dementias when the risk of financial exploitation by others may be a threat. LPAs can be registered as soon as they are drawn up. See: *www.gov.uk/power-of attorney/overview*

MEDICATION – at the early stages of dementia, medication for the condition may be prescribed. It can be effective in maintaining a quality of life. Medication comes in all forms: oral liquids, tablets, eye or ear drops, injections, creams, lotions, granules, plaster patches which contain analgesia for relief of pain, injections, and suppositories.

Carers who are live-in carers will need to know, or be taught, when and how to administer medication. Keen observation will be needed to ensure the medication is swallowed. It is possible to buy small pill pots so that people can take their medication if they go out. Unwelcome side effects of the medication should be reported to the doctor.

PAT PETS – sometimes called Therapy Pets, which are brought into a care home for residents to stroke or cuddle. It has been shown that some people with dementia respond readily to these pets when ordinarily any emotion would have been lacking. Soft cuddly toys or dolls have also proved to be effective in soothing, calming, or comforting the person with dementia.

PERISTALSIS – movement of food through the body via contractions.

PICK'S DISEASE – see Frontotemporal dementia. For more information, see: *www.alzheimers.org.uk*

VASCULAR DEMENTIA – usually caused by problems in the supply of blood to the brain. For more information, see: *www.alzheimers.org.uk*

YIELD – an emotional and physical act of letting go for the greater benefit of carers and the people for whom they are caring.

YOUNG ONSET DEMENTIA – people under the age of 65 are considered as having young onset dementia.

ZERO IN – bring the attention to bear on particular problems and seek support if necessary; focus on exactly what may be causing upset and address the issue.

CHAPTER 16 — THE SHOPPING LIST

The shopping list is an outline of items that might
be helpful in the home where primary carers
are looking after the individual with dementia.
It can serve as a checklist of necessary
things to remember such as the
necessity to organise utilities
and pay bills. Also, it reminds
carers of costs that may be
attached to some services.
There is an additional,
shorter list relating
to care homes.

Primary carers need not feel compelled to buy expensive items or products advertised in magazines that profess to make people's lives easier. Many of the mobility items can be hired out. Consult with occupational therapists for advice. The shopping list includes:

Baby alarm
Bath chair*
Bed linen and towels
Bedside tables
Bibs
Bills – especially water; heating – gas, electricity
Coloured toilet seat
Commode*
Cutlery – specially designed for arthritic hands
Electronic floor mat* – optional in a person's home but is allowed in a care home after a risk assessment
Extra appropriate clothing
Food
Hand rails
Height adjustable bed with special pressure-relieving mattress*
Hoist*
Household toiletries and cleaning agents
Incontinence pads and incontinence underwear
Incontinence mats for use on the bed and on the chairs
Mobile hairdresser
Nappy sacks
Nightwear
Patient transfer equipment such as for moving from chair to bed and vice versa
Personal toiletries
Petrol
Pressure cushions
Pressure relieving mattress*/cushions*
Sensor lights
Slippers – fitted, washable and preferably with Velcro fastening
Stair lift if the house is large enough and it can be accommodated
Stand aid*
Trips to the optician/GP/chiropodist/dentist
Tumble dryer
Underwear (ordinary)
Wages for care staff
Wages for builders and for services if the main caregiver is contemplating making adjustments to the home
Walk-in bath/shower/wet room
Walking stick
Washable mattress*
Washable waterproof mattress cover
Washable waterproof pillowcases
Washing machine
Wheelchair*
Zimmer frame* or wheelie/rollator/walkers*

*Some of these items may be loaned or provided indefinitely depending on the location and the health authority. Check on the returns procedure for loaned items. They will need removal when no longer needed especially as they may become a hazard.

In the care home

Possible additional items, which may involve a fee:

Chiropodist or podiatrist
Contribution towards outings, in-house events and entertainment
Extra meals including teas and coffees for visitors
Fees
Hairdresser
Specialist attendance such as masseur, hand care, dance and movement classes, art therapy, activity organiser